The International Development of Health Psychology

The International Development of Health Psychology

Edited by

Mary A. Jansen
Alcohol, Drug Abuse, and Mental Health Administration
United States Department of Health and Human Services
Washington, DC

and

John Weinman
The Medical School, Guy's Hospital
University of London

harwood academic publishers
chur • reading • paris • philadelphia • tokyo • melbourne

Harwood Academic Publishers

Post Office Box 90
Reading, Berkshire RG1 8JL
United Kingdom

58, rue Lhomond
75005 Paris
France

5301 Tacony Street, Drawer 330
Philadelphia, Pennsylvania 19137
United States of America

3-14-9, Okubo
Shinjuku-ku, Tokyo 169
Japan

Private Bag 8
Camberwell, Victoria 3124
Australia

Chapters 1,2,4,6,8,9,10, and 15 were originally published in Volume 4, issue 1. Chapter 7 was originally published in Volume 3, issue 2 and Chapter 13 was originally published in Volume 2, issue 4 of the journal *Psychology and Health*.

Library of Congress Cataloging-in-Publication Data

The International development of health psychology / edited by Mary A. Jansen and John Weinman.
p. cm.
Includes index.
ISBN 3-7186-5119-X
1. Clinical health psychology. 2. Clinical health psychology-Cross-cultural studies. I. Jansen, Mary A. II. Weinman, John.
[DNLM: 1. Health Education. 2. Psychology, Educational--rends.
WA 590 1606]
R726.7.I54 1991
610'.1'9--c20
DNLM/DLC 91-7019
for Library of Congress CIP

 Printed in the United States by Braun-Brumfield, Inc.

CONTENTS

Section 3: Health Psychology Training for Other Health Professionals

Section 4: Concluding Overview

INTRODUCTION

This book began life as a recent special issue of *Psychology and Health*, that was edited by Mary Jansen, Gerda Methorst and Ad Kerkhof, and described a number of international developments and approaches to training in health psychology. Since there has been a great deal of interest in this subject, we decided to extend the issue and produce this book. In doing so, we recognised that the special issue had been quite selective, therefore seven more chapters have been added in order to provide a more complete picture.

The contributions in the book are divided into four sections, each dealing with a particular theme. The first section provides overviews of the status of health psychology in a range of countries. Appropriately for the first chapter, George Stone presents a historical background to the development of the discipline, together with a summary of its progress in most regions of the world. He identifies a number of themes and factors which provide a context for understanding what has happened and what is likely to happen. Following this, René Diekstra describes another potentially important opportunity for health psychology in the World Health Organization's recommendations for primary prevention, which emphasise the role of psychological factors in health and health care. The next four papers in this section provide insights into the current standing of health psychology in a number of countries. Lothar Schmidt and Gabriele Dlugosch describe and compare the situation in a selection of European countries with quite diverse health care systems. Brian Oldenburg and Neville Owen trace a number of interesting developments in research, clinical practice and teaching in Australia. Fanny Cheung examines the beginnings of health psychology in four Chinese societies in Asia, where traditional Chinese medicine and Western medicine now coexist. She discusses some key issues in health behaviour and health care among Chinese people as a basis for understanding the slowly emerging role of health psychology. In the last paper in this section, Sølvi Kristiansen and Kerstin Søderstrøm describe the contributions of psychologists in the Cuban health care system, where emphasis is given to preventive and community-based approaches within primary health care settings.

The second section of the book examines a number of important aspects of training within health psychology. Good training will be vital in facilitating health psychology's development both as a discipline and as a profession. This training needs to begin at the undergraduate level so that psychology undergraduates can be exposed to concepts, themes and findings in health psychology. Thomas Dorsel and Andrew Baum outline the progress that has been made in undergraduate health psychology teaching in the United States and define the requirements for a basic course at this level. The next two papers deal with contrasting areas of postgraduate training, with Cynthia Belar discussing key issues in training clinical health psychologists and Stan Maes and France Kittel focusing on strategies in the training of research health psychologists. Although research and practice are often segregated in psychology, in health psychology then can and should coexist successfully, and the common theme in these two chapter provides confirmation of this. The final chapter in this section presents the data from an international survey conducted by Gerda Methorst, Mary Jansen and Ad Kerkhof. It highlights the great variety of current training approaches as well as the relatively underdeveloped situation in countries outside North America.

In the third section of the book there is a consideration of the contribution of health psychology in the training of other health professionals. Health psychology cannot exist in a vacuum in health care systems, and it is apparent that effective training of other health professional groups will facilitate health psychology's own development as well as the more widespread use of psychological approaches in different health care settings. The three papers in this section focus on training initiatives with different groups. Hal Swerrison and Peter Foreman consider the relevance of health psychology training for allied health professionals and suggest a framework for future developments. Following this, Helen Winefield discusses some fundamental issues in teaching health psychology to medical students and emphasises the need for courses to cover both basic and applied areas of the subject. In the last paper, John Christensen and Wendy Levinson report an initiative in which health psychology approaches have been incorporated into the training of medical residents. They not only describe the content areas that are covered but consider the strategies, barriers and solutions in making his type of teaching effective.

In the final section, there is an attempt to draw together many of the earlier themes in the book and to look to the future. First, John Weinman examines the various determinants that are likely to shape the concerns and activities of health psychologists over the next few years. Finally Mary Jansen, Gerda Methorst and Ad Kerkhof summarise the progress that has been made and make recommendations for training, emphasising the need for health psychologist to promote themselves and their discipline.

Taken together, the papers in this book provide an opportunity to compare the development and application of health psychology in contrasting countries. In most of these countries a great deal still needs to be done before health psychology can be considered to have arrived as a discipline and even more before it is considered a profession. Many of the factors that will hasten this process have been considered in this book, especially in the area of training. Some of the barriers to progress both within the discipline and within the broader health care contexts in which health psychologists need to work have been identified. By increasing awareness of these issues and by sharing ideas and experiences, we hope that this book will serve not only to document what has been achieved but also to define and determine future developments.

Mary A. Jansen
John Weinman

SECTION ONE

INTERNATIONAL DEVELOPMENTS OF HEALTH PSYCHOLOGY

CHAPTER 1

AN INTERNATIONAL REVIEW OF THE EMERGENCE AND DEVELOPMENT OF HEALTH PSYCHOLOGY

GEORGE C. STONE

Department of Psychiatry, University of California,
Center for the Social and Behavioral Sciences, 1350 Seventh Avenue,
CSBS 204, San Francisco, CA 94143, USA

This article presents an historical review of the development of the field of health psychology and traces its progress from its conceptual beginnings until the present. Events are chronicled in most regions of the world and the status of the field is given for these regions with a summary of the current activities taking place.

Three hypotheses are posited regarding the future development of the field with respect to its status in the country:

1. The identification of health psychology as a specific field has led to its expansion and development.
2. The history and status of psychology itself plays a major role in determining a country or region's receptivity to health psychology.
3. Where psychology is strong and autonomous and where health research and service is not dominated by medicine and psychiatry, health psychology will flourish.

A. INTRODUCTION AND EARLY DEVELOPMENTS

About fifteen years ago, in the United States, a new term was proposed for an emergent sphere of psychological activity. As early as 1974, the term "health psychology" was used in an internal memorandum proposing a new curriculum in psychology at the University of California, San Francisco. Although we felt that we had created a new and, to us at the time, a somewhat awkward sounding term, I have no doubt that others were independently trying out this unfamiliar juxtaposition of words, expressing once more the power of the *Zeitgeist.*

The first self-conscious use of the term "health psychology" in an organizational context in the United States was probably at a business meeting of the Section on Health Research of the Division of Psychologists in Public Service in 1977, when the choice of a name for a proposed new division of the American Psychological Association was debated. The next September, the Division of Health Psychology came into being. Five years later, in 1982, the Interamerican Congress of Psychology meeting in Quito, Ecuador, devoted a major part of its program to this newly named enterprise and at the meeting established a Task Force on Health Psychology. The First International Symposium of Health Psychology took place in La Habana, Cuba in 1984. Since then, there has been a veritable explosion of interest, worldwide, in the application of the concepts, knowledge, and skills of psychologists to problems of the health system. International and regional conferences have followed upon each other in quick succession.

How did this phenomenal efflorescene of activity come to pass? Does it mark the beginning of a major new field in psychology, or will it be a transient phenomenon, soon absorbed into existing categories of psychological endeavor? We are much too close to the events to give definitive answers to such questions. Yet, we must try to appraise our work and to discern the directions that offer the greatest promise of enduring contributions to human health and well-being. It is in the spirit of such appraisal and discernment that this paper is presented. Many persons in many countries are offering their views in this regard. Although I present here a personal perspective, I have tried to base it not only on my own participation in the process, but to incorporate some of the reflections of others published during these formative years. I attempt to look at the developments that took place just before and just after the crystallization of the concept of health psychology to gain insight into the emergence of this new field. In doing so, I have relied to a large extent on secondary sources—reviews and commentaries by specialists in particular topics and participants in various geographical/cultural areas.†

Three propositions appear to be supported by events of the past twenty years:

1. Although some of the activities now classifiable as health psychology have been practiced since long before the term came into use, its adoption has provided a major stimulus to the expansion and development of the field.

2. Receptivity to the idea of a field of health psychology is greatly influenced by the history and current status of the field of psychology in each sociocultural region where it is presented. Where it takes root, its development and the topics and activities it stresses are shaped by the existing forms of psychology.

3. In particular, vigorous growth occurs where there is a strong and autonomous psychology whose access to health research and services is not dominated by medicine or psychiatry.

B. RECOGNITION THAT THERE IS A FIELD OF HEALTH PSYCHOLOGY

Engaging in an activity, recognizing that we are doing so, and naming the activity are often separated by long time spans in the lives of individuals and in the history of humankind. One uses subjects and predicates long before one knows what they are. A search of Psychological Abstracts using subject headings and title words for articles about health psychology, (however labelled) turned up an average of three per year for the period from 1968–1978. In the six million volume library of the University of California, the number of books with publication dates in that period

† I wrote to a number of persons active in promoting international organizations in health psychology asking for their help in identifying the kinds of material I was seeking. Some of them sent me valuable publications. I am particularly indebted to Stan Maes of the Netherlands, Brian Oldenburg, Neville Owens, and Rob Sanson-Fisher of Australia, Andrew Steptoe and John Weinman of Great Britain and Barbara Marin of the USA. Helpful information was also received from Professor A. Appels of the Netherlands, Irmelda Florin of the Federal Republic of Germany, and Stephen Weiss of the USA.

averaged eight. But suddenly, in 1979, the year after the formation of the Division of Health Psychology and the second year following the seminal Yale Conference on Behavioral Medicine, the number of publications increased dramatically. From 1980 through 1987 the number of articles averaged 19 and the number of books, 24. It is my aim to give an overview of how this change came about and to see if we can discern from the trends of these two decades what may lie ahead. In order to achieve this, we must consider the relationships between the new field called "health psychology" and several closely related domains.

C. SOME DEFINITIONS

We begin with a definition of the field of "health psychology" proposed by Joseph Matarazzo and adopted with minor revisions by the Division of Health Psychology of the American Psychological Association in 1980. As revised, the definition reads:

> Health psychology is the aggregate of the specific educational, scientific, and professional contributions of the discipline of psychology to the promotion and maintenance of health, the prevention and treatment of illness, the identification of etiologic and diagnostic correlates of health, illness and related dysfunction, and the analysis and improvement of the health care system and health policy formation.

Interpretation of this definition requires definitions of psychology and its contributions. An earlier historical reflection proposed that psychology meant "the scientific study of the nature and determinants of human experience and behavior and the application of the knowledge thus gained in professional practice." (Rodin and Stone, 1987, p. 15). Based upon that definition, the task here can be defined as tracing the recent development of ideas about the ways in which human behavior and experience influence health and are influenced by it and of interventions based upon those ideas.

Some of these developments have appeared under the explicit label of "health psychology", and some in closely related rubrics, such as "clinical psychology", "medical psychology", "behavioral medicine", or "psychosomatics". As others have noted (Agras, 1982; Dahme and Scheer, 1984; Rodriguez, 1988; Wisocki, *et al*, 1982) it isn't possible to give a precise description of the relationships among these several categories, since definitions vary from place to place and from time to time. Nevertheless, I venture here some broadly brushed distinctions that provide a basis for bounding the phenomenon that this paper attempts to describe.

Clinical Psychology

The field first to establish itself as a domain of research and practice was clinical psychology. Throughout most of its history, clinical psychology has concerned itself almost entirely with a limited class of problems—those in which the behavior of the patient was in some sense the essence of the problem. Garfield's authoritative definition of clinical psychology as "that branch of psychology which is concerned with problems of personality adjustment and modification" (Garfield, 1965, p. 125), sounds almost as broad as those of health psychology and behavioral medicine. published more that a decade later. But almost all of the actual work performed concerned such "mental health" problems as psychosis, neurosis, and the like, problems of intellectual and emotional development, and those of alcoholism and other drugs that produced serious behavioral consequences. Mastery of techniques of assessment and treatment appropriate for these problems achieved the status of definitional characteristics of the clinical psychologist.

What now appears to have been a kind of overspecialization was pointed out in 1969 in a landmark paper (Schofield, 1969) that was a turning point for health psychology. At first, those associated with the newly identified field of health research, as it was called during the first formative years, made much of the distinction of their new endeavor from the traditional problems of Clinical Psychology, even though many of the participants were clinical psychologists by training. In recent years, with the concept of a health psychology firmly established, this sharp distinction is, quite properly, being softened and much of the present growth in health psychology is occurring as an expansion and broadening of long-standing programs in clinical psychology. As this process continues, a major region of health psychology will be oriented to work with emotional and intellectual problems of persons in the health care phase of the health system.

Psychosomatics

Even earlier than the application of psychology to mental health problems, were the beginnings of a theoretical concern with the role of psychological factors in the etiology of bodily disease. The term "psychosomatic medicine" was coined in 1818 by a German named Heinroth to describe his concern with the role of internal conflict in causing mental disease (Wittkower, 1974). Vigorous work in the application of psychoanalytic theory to the understanding of certain physical diseases began in Germany during the 1920's and came to the United States with Franz Alexander about 1930 and to England in 1933 in the person of Eric Wittkower. Psychosomatics has also been long established and well developed in a number of other countries. The concept of psychosomatic diseases reached its peak in the 1940's and early 50's. Then increasing methodological rigor revealed that the relationships were more general and less symbolically colorful than the early workers had portrayed them. The term "psychosomatic medicine" persists to refer to a special emphasis on holism and on symbolic influences within the body of behavioral medicine.

Medical Psychology

The term "medical psychology" has been used in quite different ways in different times and places. In Great Britain it has been essentially synonymous with "psychiatry'. Throughout much of Europe (Dahme and Scheer, 1986; Predescu and Ionescu, 1972, Shostakovich, 1968) and parts of Latin America (Castro-Gonzalo, 1973) it has referred to psychological aspects of the curative interactions between physicians and their patients. Most of what has been published about this topic in the past quarter of a century concerns teaching medical students and professionals to appreciate the need for a humanistic and holistic approach to patients' problems. It incorporates material from psychomatics (Asken, 1979; Dahme and Scheer, 1984), doctor-patient relationships (Castro-Gonzalo, 1973, Predescu and Ionesco, 1972) and ethics and humanism (Lobo, 1986).

Behavioral Medicine

Behavioral medicine is that part of the field of medicine that seeks to accomplish its objectives through behavioral means. Clearly, this definition gains specificity only when the objectives of medicine have been spelled out. These specifications have been the subject of a good deal of discussion and controversy. A formal definition of behavioral medicine, comparable in scope to Matarazzo's definition of health psychology given above, was adopted at the Yale Conference on Behavioral Medicine in 1977. In the following year, at a conference sponsored by the United States' National Academy of Science's Institute of Medicine, the definition was refined to stress the integration of concepts and practices from the biomedical and the behavioral antecedents:

Behavioral medicine is the interdisciplinary field concerned with the development and integration of behavioral and biomedical science knowledge techniques relevant to health and illness and the application of this knowledge and these techniques to prevention, diagnosis, treatment, and rehabilitation. (Schwartz and Weiss, 1978).

In many parts of the world, the amended Yale definition has provided the reference point against which alternatives could be measured (Alcaraz and Diaz de Leon, 1985; Biondi, 1983; Inglis, 1983; Schreurs, Winnubst, Kruithof and Willige, 1984). Gentry (1984) attributes the first use of the term "behavioral medicine" to a book edited by Birk (1973) titled *Biofeedback: Behavioral Medicine.* The context implies a much narrower definition: behavioral medicine equals biofeedback. This view has not persisted, however. One of the commonest alternative versions places heavy emphasis on behavioral techniques derived from conditioning theory. (Brockway 1978; Pomerleau 1979). This viewpoint has been favored in some of the Latin American countries (Rodriguez and Blanca, 1983) and has advocates in Europe, as well (Fanchon, 1983).

How does health psychology relate to the Yale conception of behavioral medicine? Within the conceptual domain of health psychology as set forth above there are psychologists trained to carry out, among them, many of the research or practice interventions of behavioral medicine. But there are also relevant interventions of anthropologists, sociologists, economists, etc. that constitute a part of the armamentarium of behavioral medicine. Physicians and other medical workers can learn to perform many of these interventions through post-graduate education or can work in close collaboration with behavioral scientists in doing so. In many instances it is the intimate association of the behavioral and nonbehavioral interventions in treating illness that gives behavioral medicine its distinctive character. It should be clear that much of health psychology consists of psychologists doing things included within the domain of behavioral medicine, if the Yale definition, or one equally broad, is accepted.

To summarize then, and return the discussion to the more focused field of health psychology, it can be asserted that in the broadest sense, health psychology encompasses any scientific or professional application of psychological concepts or methods to any problem arising in the health system, not only the care giving system, but the public health, health education, health planning, health financing, health legislation and other such components of the total system (Stone, 1979, 1988). Under this view, any branch of psychology that deals with the health system would be a subdivision of health psychology. Thus, the traditional practice of clinical psychology, which focuses on mental health problems, would be such a subdivision. So would neuropsychology and rehabilitation psychology. From an organizational point of view it doesn't make sense to subordinate older, larger, better defined enterprises to one hardly more than a decade old; but conceptually, the relations with other fields can be seen more simply if this grouping is recognized. Then we can recognize that health psychology (as a whole) overlaps with an interdisciplinary field of application, such as behavioral medicine, and also with public health, health promotion, rehabilitation, etc., to a greater or lesser degree as psychologists have found ways to apply their knowledge and skills to the issues of those fields.

But considerable differences exist in different parts of the world with respect to use of the terms "health psychology" and "behavioral medicine". Persual of the international literature suggests that pre-existing conditions have a causal effect in the adoption of one of these terms, and that adoption of one or both has a substantial impact on the amount and type of work that is done. A discussion of the international differences follows.

D. NATIONAL EMPHASES IN THE DEVELOPMENT OF HEALTH PSYCHOLOGY

It is not possible here to present even brief sketches of the situation in each of the countries for which information is available. I have therefore selected examples of several patterns of development to support three hypotheses I have gleaned about major factors that are influential. These are:

1. As psychologists have discovered the relevance of their theory and techniques to problems of the health system, the form taken by their applications is very strongly shaped by the existing state of psychology as a discipline and a profession in their country.
2. The adoption of the term "health psychology" to describe the application of psychological theory and practice to health problems has had an invigorating and focusing effect on psychologists engaged in the enterprise.
3. The choice of this term as opposed to some others such as "medical psychology" or "behavioral medicine" has been facilitated in those countries where there is already a strong and independent profession of psychology.

In describing the patterns of development which follow, I have relied on reports and discussions of work I call "health psychology", regardless of who has carried it out or what they may have called it. The patterns described are not well organized geographically as two neighboring countries may reflect dissimilar developments, each of them with developments similar to those of one or more countries on another continent.

A particularly strong example of regionalization with a very stimulating effect is in Latin America, due to the formative influence of the Interamerican Society of Psychology (ISP). Formed in 1951, meeting biennally since 1953, and publishing the well circulated journals *Revista Latinoamericana de Psicologia* and the Interamerican Psychologist (Psicologo Interamericano—presented bilingually), this organization has promoted continuing contact among psychologists throughout the Americas. As soon as the identities of behavioral medicine and health psychology began to take shape, they found a place on the programs of the Interamerican meetings. The Task Force on Health Psychology was formed in 1982 which has been assiduously promoting communication among psychologists in the various nations of the Americas ever since (Marin and Donovan, 1988).

Patterns in the Developed World

(a) Countries with an extended tradition of basic research in health psychology. The first pattern to be put forward is that of a country in which there has long been an active interest in research on specific and focal relationships between psychological processes and health issues. The research is quite basic, and in the forefront of international progress. An outstanding example of this pattern is Sweden.

The development of health psychology in Sweden has been dominated by the psychophysiological studies of stress at the Karolinska Institute in Stockholm. Beginning in the early 1970s, Levi (1972) and Frankenhauser (1975) began important long term projects to characterize how people react to the stress of a normal environment—on the job, riding public transit, children in daycare, adjustment to retirement are just a few examples. This work, influenced by and interacting with the sociopolitical context in Sweden, has produced a strong emphasis on locating stressors in the physical and social environment and in seeking to eliminate them through legislative and administrative initiatives. There has been substantial research and application of findings in the areas of work psychology, including the effects of shift work schedules, job demands in terms of pace, monotony, and decision latitude. Other topics related to the stress area have also been the subject of research—social support, cardiovascular epidemiology (studies of Type A behavior). As noted, there is a rather strong emphasis on public health and social policy approaches in intervention. Some Swedes as well as outside critics have raised the question whether there has not been a relative neglect of the characteristics of individual persons as factors influencing health and of interventions directed to individuals (Theorell, 1986).

Other candidates for mention in this category would include Russia, where Pavlovian psychophysiology has been applied to a range of problems, and several other countries—Germany, England, Finland, Italy, and perhaps Spain—where psychosomatic theory has been tested, if not with great rigor, against empirical observations; and countries like Finland where a theoretical but methodologically sophisticated epidemiology has been applied to psychosocial factors in health.

(b) Countries in which clinical applications dominate. Perhaps the best exemplar of this pattern is Great Britain. In Great Britain clinical psychology is integrated to a large degree into the general medical services. Although this situation may promote effective contributions to health care, it seems to be perceived as retarding the development of a vigorous and independent field of health psychology in Great Britain. Steptoe and Moses (1986) comment that "behavioral scientists remain 'poor relations' in many medical schools and research centers." At another point in their review of psychosocial research on health problems, these authors comment on the close integration of work on etiology and intervention resulting in what amounts to a "clinical bias" even in experimental studies. The concern expressed by Marteau and Johnston (1987) that health psychology in general may be suffering from an insufficiency of theoretical models, may be influenced by these same factors.

From an organizational point of view, both the clinical emphasis and integration, and the problems with funding mechanisms and level, also reported by Steptoe and Moses (1986), may constitute obstacles to the development of health psychology in Great Britain. From a trans-Atlantic perspective, there does not appear to be any shortage of influence in the world's literature nor any failure of participation in the international movement toward interchange and cooperation by psychologists in Great Britain. There does seem to be a surprising lack of contact between the internationally outstanding British work in experimental, cognitive, and ergonomic psychology and the health domain. British contributions to health psychology have thus far been predominantly to the interpersonal aspects of health care and to an enriching of our understanding of patients' experiences in the health care system and to physicians' response to patients (e.g. Balint and Norell, 1973; Calnan, 1987; Gillis, 1972).

Two quite different variants on this pattern are to be found in Norway and Australia (Ursin, 1986; Oldenburg and Owen, this issue). In Norway, where behavioral medicine is being shaped by a relative absence of psychologists from medical school teaching faculties, a strong independent profession of psychology is growing up, emphasizing brain research and neuropsychology (Ursin, 1986). Australiàn health psychology, as detailed by Oldenburg and Owen (this issue), has achieved substantial responsibility in the education of health professionals and has developed a strongly behavioral approaches to clinical interventions.

(c) Countries with a medically oriented emphasis on teaching. In several countries the contact between psychology and the problems of the health system has been primarily through teaching physicians-in-training about the psychology of the patient and the doctor-patient interaction. To exemplify this pattern, I chose the Federal Republic of Germany, even though it is presently undergoing a rapid transition into the contemporary, broad spectrum form of health psychology/behavioral medicine.

The term "medical psychology" continues to be preferred in West Germany. Almost all of the literature citations I found from this country made use of that term. Appropriately, in discussing definitions and distinctions, Dahme and Scheer (1986) establish their subject as "the application of psychological concepts and methods to medical problems." A journal, *Medizinische Psychologie*, was established in 1974, and the term was introduced in Germany nearly 150 years ago by Lotze (Dahme and Scheer, 1986, p. 19).

In the Federal Republic of Germany, as in East Germany, Austria, France, and Argentina, the primary role of medical psychologists has been the teaching of medical students. In such teaching, major points of emphasis have been the psychology of the patient, the stresses of the medical and hospital environments and of dealing with severe and chronic illness, and especially, with physician-patient interactions. In both research and practice, German psychologists have concentrated on assisting patients in dealing with the stresses of their illnesses and treatments, and in assisting physicians in their efforts to provide the best care through supporting their diagnoses and decision-making, improving their understanding of patients and their needs, and enhancing the quality of the doctor-patient interactions. Although, according to Dahme and Scheer (1986), much of this work is theoretically undergirded by the writings of Janis and the Lazarus group, impressively reviewed for German readers by Davies-Osterkamp (1982), it appears that the attention being given to these issues in a wide variety of medical situations and settings in West Germany during the 1980's exceeds that originating in the United States.

More recently, a Deutsche Gesellschaft für Verhaltensmedizin und Verhaltensmodifikation (German Association of Behavioral Medicine and Behavior Modification) was formed in 1984. It had about 150 members in the fall of 1988, about a fourth of whom are physicians. The first congress of this organization was held in

March, 1987 in Munich. Discussions are currently being held to consider whether federal funding of a research program in health psychology should be inaugurated. So far, it appears, the sentiment for a very interdisciplinary approach is strong and "it has not been well defined in which aspects behavioral medicine differs from health psychology" (Florin, personal communication).

(d) Countries where there have been recent upsurges of vigorous activity displacing older patterns. Mention has already been made of the rapid expansion of contemporary research in the Federal Republic of Germany. Similar changes are occurring in the Netherlands, Italy and Japan. A particularly interesting transition has been occurring in Spain. There is available a very thoughtful interpretation of developments written by a Spanish psychiatrist (Lobo, 1986) and several written by psychologists actively participating in research, clinical work, and the establishment of training programs for health psychologists (Fernandez-Ballesteros and Carrobles 1988; Reig, Rodriguez and Mira, 1987). The picture is one of a rich philosophical tradition being challenged by a vigorous new brand of health psychology strong in both its theoretical and its clinical emphases. As was said of work in Great Britain, research is closely tied to practice, with substantial amounts of work being conducted on a wide range of topics, from pain control (Labrador, Vallejo, and Cruzado, 1986) and the placebo effect (Perez and Martinez, 1987) to psychological cofactors in AIDS (Bayes and Arranz, 1988). Cross-cultural, international collaboration has been established with health psychologists in Mexico to conduct comparative epidemiological studies on university populations and to compare the effectiveness of behavioral treatments in the two countries (Bayes, Riba, Seligson, Lizeaga, Riveros, Silva, and Nava, 1987). Of four post-doctoral training programs existing in 1987 in Europe, two were in Spain, at Madrid and Valencia.

Fernandez-Ballesteros and Carrobles (1988) provide information that could help to account for such a high level of activity. The Spanish constitution, adopted in 1978, declares that health is a right of Spanish citizens and specifies in some detail how it is to be protected and preserved. These declarations have been backed up more recently by laws and administrative procedures that place high priority on health and industrial hygiene. A second factor appears to be the strong organizations of psychologists that exist in the various provinces in Spain—organizations that both cooperate and also compete for preeminence. Lobo (1986) makes reference to a pervasive "feeling of generalized inferiority" among Spanish intellectuals dating back into the nineteenth century. He now sees this mood as "quickly disappearing," a change that is surely warranted by the important contributions of Spanish health psychologists.

Patterns in the Developing World

(a) Developing countries with westernized elites. A number of countries have been attempting to overcome the various factors that have impeded their full development by modeling their societies predominantly after those of the technological leaders of the West. Quite a range of development in the area of health psychology is to be found among them. In Greece, emerging from a long and difficult period of post-war recovery and development, clinical psychology is barely getting started, and there is as yet no sign of health psychology (Bouhoutsos and Roe, 1984). Mexico, by

contrast, in spite of severe economic difficulties, has a strongly developed applied psychology, and health psychology is beginning to be established across a broad spectrum.

A midrange, and instructive example is found in Egypt. David (1965) described a situation in that country with a fairly well developed role for clinical psychologists existing 25 years ago in 1965. There were some "properly trained" professional psychologists, mostly educated in Great Britain or the United States, although they were "overwhelmed with demands for clinical services." There was an established Egyptian Psychological Association that took a strong interest in the development of psychological services and the establishment of professional standards. As early as 1956 there was a law stipulating the conditions and qualifications for the practice of psychotherapy. In spite of these promising circumstances, as of a recent report, "no psychologists with Ph.D.'s are on the faculties of medical schools. Teaching and research are currently dominated by medical doctors, mainly in psychiatry." (Ashour, 1986, p. 19). According to this open-minded psychiatrist, behavioral medicine is barely beginning, the skills of psychologists are badly needed in psychiatry departments, and "these Ph.D.'s should learn to live and work with psychiatrists."

(b) Developing countries with strong commitments to community development. In developing countries where centralized planning for health care has predominated, the concept of health psychology appeared early and its approach tended to be community-oriented. A very successful instance of this form of development in Cuba has been ably documented by the person who established a group of health psychologists in 1969 and directed it for many years (Garcia-Averasturi 1980, 1985). A special issue of the *Journal of Community Psychology*, devoted to the topic of community psychology in Cuba (Bernal and Marin, 1985) provides much additional background.

The small Central American country of Costa Rica was able to elaborate at an early point a comprehensive plan for a prevention/development oriented, community-based program for its fully socialized health care system (Ruphuy, 1977). The plan grew out of a new curriculum adopted by the faculty of medicine at the University of Costa Rica aimed at engaging physicians in the national problems of underdevelopment and health. The training was intended to develop physicians who understood and were able to work with behavioral scientists. Along with this program of medical training, a program for training "intermediate professionals" in psychology was developed. In this five-year program, these individuals were to be trained primarily to work as change agents, returning as far as possible to the communities from which they had come and using their broadly conceived education in the social and behavioral sciences to advise the community health teams in efforts to motivate, educate and support community members in attacking their own problems of health and community development.

The situation prior to the Ruphuy report may be seen from an article describing medical psychology as "an orientation which emphasizes the bio-psycho-social unity of man" or as a "set of attitudes present in the doctor-patient relationship" (Castro-Gonzalo, 1973). This fairly typical European viewpoint was published with French and German, but not English, summaries. Descriptions of the health care process based on observations made by anthropologists at about the time when Ruphuy's paper was published (Low, 1982; data from 1973) and about ten years later

(Hill, 1985) suggest that neither the European ideal nor the community-based model were widely practiced.

A third country that could be mentioned as exemplifying the community-oriented approach is India. Because traditional beliefs have been such an important (and discussed) factor in implementing health programs there, it might have been mentioned also in the following category. There has been a strong commitment in India to planned change that would "telescope the process of development" (Sinha 1988). Health issues have been cast to a considerable degree within the context of "healthy human development" and there has been strong emphasis on the role of the family in mitigating the stresses and accomplishing the goals of rapid social change. Concepts of behavioral medicine are also taking root, emphasizing the use of behavior modification in approaching health problems (Kaushik, 1985).

(c) Developing countries with very different conceptions of health processes. I have been attempting to demonstrate that health psychology develops in a particular context as a kind of overlay on the psychology already present in that context. In countries where Euro/American psychology has not yet taken a firm hold, concepts of health assume a larger role in determining the kind of health psychology that takes shape. This factor is important in many Latin American countries and its influence in India has already been noted.

The developing countries in Africa are hardly yet in a position to participate fully in the international development of health psychology as there are very few psychologists there and those that are there are preoccupied with very basic issues. A rich and sensitive portrayal of African views of mind-body relationships has been provided by Ebigo (1986). In much of black Africa, according to this writer, physical and mental illness are generally attributed to disordered relationships with spirits or sorcerers, including those brought on by the breaking of taboos. Such beliefs, coupled with prevalent child-rearing practices create a situation in which the somatization of emotional distress is nearly universal. And severe stress is endemic as a result of cultural conflict arising when demands for modernization clash with deeply held traditions. The strong commitments to the group that characterize village life in Africa create needs for learning about the possibility of individual autonomy and responsibility that are vital for successful integration into contemporary industrial, urban settings. But there is also much to be learned from a reconsideration by Westerners of the important influences of the group, which may contribute to the transition to a post-industrial world culture. As psychological procedures are brought to bear on health issues in these countires, a socio/developmental emphasis will be critically important.

E. SUMMARY

This article has attempted to examine the introduction and adoption of a new specialization "health psychology" to describe a field of scientific and professional activity that applied the concepts, knowledge, and techniques of psychology to problems of the health system. It has attempted to determine whether the use of this term, as opposed to others used to describe closely related bodies of work, has had an influence on the developing patterns of research and practice engaged in by those who think of themselves as health psychologists.

I can hardly offer conclusions from this survey as scientifically warranted facts. There does appear to be a pattern that I have offered more as an interpretation to be verified than as something already demonstrated.

The story, to recapitulate it in its briefest form, goes as follows: For many years—as long as there have been psychologists—there have been efforts to apply psychology to phenomena of health, illness, and health care. At first these attempts were neither intense nor extensive, and they were not distinguished by any particular labels. Mostly they took the form of proposing curricula and, sometimes, participating in the teaching of medical students or physicians about the "human aspects of medicine." When clinical psychology began to take shape, some of its viewpoints and techniques were applied by psychologists whose work brought them unto contact with physicians and patients outside of the mental health facilities where most clinical psychologists worked. Some psychophysiologists and some psychodynamic theorists did research on the etiology of diseases. A few social psychologists studied attitudes about health and illness and tried to apply their theories to communications intended to promote the adoption of behaviors favorable to health. To the degree that work of this kind was recognized as anything special, it was described as "psychology in medicine" or "medical psychology." Those who engaged in it were seen as expatriates, working as aliens in foreign lands.

Suddenly, in the last years of the 1960s, a number of psychologists noticed that there were vast territories in the health system that were psychologically underdeveloped. In the United States, they began to communicate and to organize, and after a half decade they had coined or discovered the terms "behavioral medicine" and "health research" to describe what they were doing. Among their numbers were some who argued that "behavioral medicine" was not a sufficient rubric under which to expand the role of psychologists in the health system, since it seemed to perpetuate the medical dominance that had relegated most psychologists to second class citizenship in the health care system. "Medical psychology" had some of the same drawbacks. It was also argued that this outbreak of psychological activity in the health system should not and would not be limited to research, but would involve professional interventions at the level of individual patients, their families, health care providers and organizations. Finally, psychological viewpoints influenced already by the biopsychosocial model and by traditions from community, social, and humanistic psychology that placed substantial emphasis on the prevention of illness and the promotion of health, supported the use of the word "health" in the name of the emerging enterprise to underscore these views. Thus the term "health psychology" was adopted in 1977 as the title under which this group would set out to establish a new field in psychology.

At first, most of the work of health psychologists was in the interdisciplinary medical settings where behavioral medicine took place. As more and more psychologists came to think of themselves as health psychologists the scope of their activities broadened. Also, they increasingly perceived that their influence in medical settings would be strengthened if they came with a clear and respected disciplinary identity of their own. Instead of being expatriates, they would become second and third generation members of a valued subgroup in the medical world. Thus, in the past few years, it appears that health psychology and behavioral medicine are growing side by side. Health psychology is a broader field than behavioral medicine, in terms of the range of the problems and settings that occupy its attention; behavioral medicine is home to scientists and practitioners from a number of disciplines in addition to psychology. The relationship between them should not be competitive, but harmonious and cooperative.

The future of health psychology will be one of continued growth and productivity if we emphasize two themes among the many that can be found in our short history. First, we should devote our efforts to bringing more and more of the theory and practice of all of psychology to bear on problems of the entire health system. In so doing we will create a broad base for an autonomous science/profession whose special capabilities will gain wide recognition. Second, we should develop our ability to see the health system not only as a place in which we can offer immediate service but as a rich source of settings for the validation and extension of our principles and procedures. We need to enhance our capacity to engage both the patients/clients and the workers of the health system as participants in the discovery of new psychological knowledge and the testing of new techniques, rather than as subjects to be mystified and even exploited by a professional elite. If we are successful in this, we will gain access to psychological phenomena that cannot possibly be simulated in academic laboratories, and our research will become a major source of new knowledge for psychology as a whole. Then, health psychologists will be distinguished from other psychologists by the depth and breadth of their knowledge of health issues and of the people, organizations, and institutions that comprise the health system. Such a future can be bright indeed.

References

Agras, W. S. (1982). Behavioral medicine in the 1980s: Nonrandom connections. *Journal of Consulting and Clinical Psychology,* **50**, 797–803.

Alcaraz, V. M. and Diaz de Leon, A. E. (1985). New behavioral approaches to disease. In Juan Jose Sanchez-Sosa (Ed.), *Health and Clinical Psychology*. (pp. 585–596). North-Holland: Elsevier Science Publishers.

Ashour, A. M. (1986). Mind-body disease investigations in Egypt: A psychiatrist's monopoly. *Advances,* **3**(4), 15–18.

Asken, M. J. (1979). Medical psychology: Toward definition, clarification and organization. *Professional Psychology,* **10**(1), 66–73.

Balint, E. and Norell, J. S. (Eds.). (1973). *Six minutes for the patient; interactions in general practice consultation*. London: Tavistock Publications.

Bayes, R. and Arranz, P. (1988). Las variables psicologicas como cofactores del sindrome de immunodificiencia adquiritda. *JANO: Medicina y Humanidades,* **34**(812), 32–42.

Bayes, R., Riba, M. D., Seligson, I., Lizeaga, N., Riveros, G., Silva, A., and Nava, C. (1987). *Un estudio transcultural sobre alqunos trastornos de salud en poblaciones universitarias: Su importancia para la investigacion y didactica de las terapia conductuales*. Paper presented at the 21st Interamerican Congresss of Psychology, La Habana, Cuba, June 28–July 3, 1987.

Bernal, G. and Marin, B. (Eds.). (1985). Community psychology in Cuba. *Journal of Community Psychology,* **13**(2), Whole.

Biondi, M. (1983). Medicina comportamental: Epidemiologia, prevenzione e terapia per le malattie sometiche. *Revista de Psichiatria* **18**(2), 91–132.

Birk, L. (Ed.) (1973). *Biofeedback: Behavioral Medicine*. New York: Grune and Stratton.

Bouhoustos, J. C. and Roe, K. V. (1984, January). Mental health services and the emerging role of psychology in Greece. *American Psychologist,* **39**(1), 57–61.

Brockway, B. S. (1978). Behavioral medicine in family practice: A unifying approach for the assessment and treatment of psychosocial problems. *Southern Journal of Family Practice.* **6**(3), 545–552.

Calnan, M. (1987). *Health and illness: The lay perspective.* New York: Tavistock Publications.

Castro-Gonzalo, A. (1973). Psychological aspects of the practice of medicine. *Revista de Neuro-Psiquiatria,* **36**(4), 260–267.

Dahme, B. and Scheer, J. W. (1984). Medical psychology. *German Journal of Psychology,* **8**(2), 138–180.

Dahme, B. and Scheer, J. W. (1986). Medical psychology in the Federal Republic of Germany. *Advances,* **3**(4), 19–35.

David, H. (1965). International trends in clinical psychology. In Wolman, B. E. (Ed.) *Handbook of Clinical Psychology*. New York: McGraw Hill.

Davies-Osterkamp, S. (1982). Angst und angstbewaltigung bei chirugischen patienten. In Beckmann D., Davies-Osterkamp S., Scheer J. W., (Eds.). *Medizinische Psychologie*. Berlin: Springer-Verlag.

Ebigo, P. (1986). The mind, the body and society: An African perspective. *Advances,* **3**(4), 45–57.

Fanchon, L. (1983). Medecine comportementale et psychologie de la sante. *International Review of Applied Psychology,* **32**(2), 183–197.

Fernandez-Ballesteros, R. and Carrobles, J. A. (1988). Perspectivas de la psicologia de la salud en Europa. *Psicologos Papeles del Colegio,* **6**(33/34), 3–11.

Frankenhauser, M. (1975). Sympathetic-adrenomedullary activity, behaviour, and the psychosocial environment. In P. H. Venables and M. J. Christie (Eds.), *Research in Psychophysiology*. New York: Wiley.

Garcia-Averasturi, L. (1980). Psychology and health care in Cuba. *American Psychologist,* **35**, 1090–1095.

Garcia-Averasturi, L. (1985). Community health psychology in Cuba. Special issue: Community psychology in Cuba. *Journal of Community Psychology* **13**(2), 117–123.

Garfield, S. (1965). Historical introduction. In Wolman, Benjamin B. (Ed.). *Handbook of Clinical Psychology*. New York: McGraw-Hill.

Gentry, W. D. (1984). Behavioral medicine: A new research paradigm. In W. D. Gentry (Ed.) *Handbook of behavioral medicine*. New York: Guilford.

Gillis, L. (1972). Human Behavior in Illness: Psychology and Interpersonal Relationships (2nd Ed). London: Faber.

Hill, C. E. (1985). Local health knowledge and universal primary health care: A behavioral case from Costa Rica. *Medical Anthropology*. Winter, 11–23.

Inglis, J. (1983). Behavioural science and behavioural medicine revisited. *Canadian Journal of Behavioral Science*. **15**(4), 305–317.

Kaushik, S. S. (1985). From behavioural science to behaviour modification and to behavioural medicine. University Grants Commission National Seminar (1985, New Delhi, India). *Dayalbagh Educational Institute Research Journal of Education,* **3**(1), 8–12.

Labrador, F. J., Vallejo, M. A. and Cruzado, J. A. (1986). Tratamientos conductuales del dolor. *JANO: Medicina y Humanidades,* **30**(708), 44–60.

Levi, K. (Ed.) (1972). Stress and distress in response to psychosocial stimuli. *Acta Medica Scandinavica: Supplement* No. 528, Whole.

Lobo, A. (1986). Philosophical humanism and empirical science: Spanish perspectives on psychosomatics. *Advances,* **3**(4), 58–76.

Low, S. (1982). The effect of medical institutions on doctor-patient interaction in Costa Rica. *Milbank Memorial Fund Quarterly/Health and Society,* **60**(1), 17–51.

Marin, B. and David, A. (1988). A survey of health psychology in the Americas. *Interamerican Psychologist* **66**, 7–9.

Marteau, T. M. and Johnston, M. (1987). Health psychology: The danger of neglecting psychological models. *Bulletin of the British Psychological Society* **40**, 82–85.

Perez, M. and Martinez, J. (1987). Psychology of the placebo effect and basis for its international clinical use (English translation). *Estudios de Psicolgia,* **31**, 82–100.

Pomerleau, O. F. (1979). Behavioral medicine: The contribution of the experimental analysis of behavior to medical care. *American Psychologist,* **34**(8), 654–663.

Predescu, V. and Ionescu, G. (1972). Psychology: An implicit dimension of medicine. *Neurologia, Psihiatria, Neurochirurgia,* **17**(4), 290–298.

Reig, A., Rodriguez, J. and Mira, J. J. (1987). Psicologia de la salud: Algunas cuestiones basicas. *Informacio Psicologica,* **30**, 5–10.

Rodin, J. and Stone, G. (1987). Historical highlights in the emergence of the field. In G. C. Stone, S. M. Weiss, J. D. Matarazzo, *et al* (Eds.). *Health Psychology, a discipline and a profession* Chicago: The University of Chicago Press.

Rodriguez, J. (1988). Una alternativa para uno de los futuros posibles de la psicologia. *Psicologos papelas del colegio* **6**(33/34), 13–18.

Rodriguez, B. and Blanca, L. (1983). Medicina conductual: Su definicion y aplicacion. Behavioral medicine: Its definition and application. *Revista de Analisis del Comportamiento,* **1**(1), 75–91.

Ruphuy, R. S. (1977). Psychology and medicine: A new approach for community health development. *American Psychologist,* **32**(11), 910–913.

Schofield, W. (1969). The role of psychology in the delivery of health services. *American Psychologist,* **24**, 565–584.

Schreurs, P. J., Winnubst, J. A., Kruithof, W. and Willige, G. V. (1984). Behavioral Medicine: Symbiose van psychologie en geneeskunde. *Gedrag: Tijdschrift Voor Psychologie,* **12**(1–2), 3–14.

Schwartz, G. E. and Weiss, S. M. (1978). Behavioral medicine revisited: An amended definition. *Journal of Behavioral Medicine,* **1**, 249–252.

Shostakovich, V. V. (1969). Subject matter and objectives of medical psychology. *Zhurnal Nevropatologii I Psikhiatrii.* **9**, 1412–1414.

Sinha, D. (1988). The family scenario in a developing country and its implications for mental health—The case of India. In P. R. Dasen, J. W. Berry and N. Sartorious, *Health and Cross Cultural Psychology: Toward Applications.* Beverly Hills, CA: Sage.

Steptoe, A. and Moses, J. (1986). Psychosocial processes in disease: A research perspective from the United Kingdom. *Advances,* **3**(4), 83–91.

Stone, G. C. (1979). Psychology and health. In G. C. Stone, F. Cohen, N. E. Adler and Associates, *Health Psychology.* San Francisco, CA: Jossey-Bass.

Stone, G. C. (1988). Psicologia de la salud: Una definicion amplia. *Revista Latinoamericana de Psicologia,* **20**(1), 15–26.

Theorell, T. (1986). Research on stress and health in Sweden from 1950 to 1985. *Advances,* **3**(4), 92–104.

Ursin, H. (1986). Behavioral medicine in Norway. *Advances,* **3**(4), 105–113.

Wisocki, P. (1982). Definitional issues in behavioral medicine. *Scandinavian Journal of Behaviour Therapy* **11**(2), 57–63.

Wittkower, E. D. (1974). Historical perspective on contemporary psychosomatic medicine. *International Journal of Psychiatry in Medicine,* **5**(4), 309–319.

CHAPTER 2

PSYCHOLOGY, HEALTH AND HEALTH CARE

RENÉ F. W. DIEKSTRA

Department of Health Psychology, University of Leiden, Leiden, The Netherlands

This article traces the development of the World Health Organization's emphasis on psychological and behavioural factors in health and notes its encouragement of recognition of these factors by member states. The article further outlines the reasons for this increasing recognition and stresses the important role of psychological and behavioural factors in the maintenance of health and prevention of illness.

1. INTRODUCTION

The Behaviour–Health Relationship

Behaviour related chronic and disabling diseases are now the leading causes of death in the industrialized world, and they are rapidly gaining significance in the developing world, especially in the urbanized areas. But there is also a growing recognition of the role that behaviour plays in the spread and control of parasitic and infectious diseases, that have been and still are the most frequent cause of death and disability in most developing countries. Schistosomiasis or Bilharzia, for example, represents a constant threat to as many as 600 million people in the world. It has been established, as has been formulated in a recent WHO report of experts on Schistosomiasis, that the modification of the behaviour of people, urinating and defaecating in water that is also used for swimming, fishing, farming, washing and bathing, is crucial for the control or the elimination of the disease.

Individuals who are suffering from chronic diseases such as diabetes, respiratory diseases, hypertension, ischaemic heart disease, cancer and sexually transmitted diseases often have contracted or aggravated their illnesses as a result of careless, dangerous or unhealthy behaviour. Bad eating habits, abuse of alcohol and tobacco, refusal to adhere to hygiene and safety prescriptions and lack of skills in coping with life stresses are among the most salient of such behaviours.

It has also been found that such individuals have stress-related problems and emotional difficulties arising from their diseases and impaired functioning. These in turn keep them from following doctor's orders or health advice from other sources.

But it is not only through its causative role in the development, course and outcome of diseases, that behaviour takes its toll. It is often a direct cause of physical and mental disability and malfunctioning. Each year an estimated 400 million persons are injured by accidents (often involving the use of alcohol or other psychoactive substances) or by intentional violent behaviour by themselves or by others, even from their own families, serious enough to require medical attention.

Recent data show that road traffic accidents are becoming as important a cause of death in developing countries as they are already in developed countries. The same appears to be the case with self inflicted or suicidal deaths. In contrast to the past, the highest suicide rates are nowadays not found in countries in the developed, but in the developing world.

Such changes in patterns of morbidity and mortality are related to the fact that in many countries people are subject to rapid social changes, resulting from economic development, industrialization and urbanization. Because of the effect these developments have on the structure of communities and family functioning, they can often no longer cope by using their traditional ways of behaving and of solving problems.

Erosion of traditional support systems and loss of social cohesion, often aggravated by migration and uprooting, throw many into a state of alienation and anomie. They become vulnerable to the lure of alcoholism and drug abuse, or may develop such adverse emotional states as brutalization, apathy, depression or other mental health problems. There is a concomitant increase in developmental and behavioural problems in children and adolescents as well as in loneliness and accompanying emotional and health problems in the elderly.

Behaviour, Health and Health Care Systems

What effects does the situation described above have on the functioning of health care systems and the problems or disorders they have to deal with?

A recent review of the relevant literature (Diekstra, 1989) concludes that: "Studies in the industrialized countries indicate that 30–50% of all consultations are by patients who exhibit no ascertainable organ pathology, or who complain of discomfort and disfunctioning disproportionate to their physical problems. In developing countries such patients make up 20–35% of those coming to the attention of health care personnel, therewith constituting the largest single complaint category in primary health care."

According to some authors this category of patients is still growing while at the same time the number of patients with clear-cut hardboiled neuroses is gradually declining. Roughly speaking we are dealing here with two categories of patients or helpseekers. The first contains those with so called functional complaints, that is complaints implying somatic distress and symptoms unaccounted for by pathological findings, attributed by the sufferer to physical illness, who therefore seeks medical help for them (Lipowski, 1988).

Within this group one needs to distinguish between those without any underlying organ pathology, and those with ascertainable organ pathology but who present complaints or suffer from symptoms unaccounted for by that pathology, such as chronically ill patients who for one reason or another exacerbate their symptoms or disability.

The second category consists of patients—who may or may not be chronically ill—before or after surgery, who for a multitude of reasons experience distress, symptoms or complications in excess to what can be expected or explained by their pre- or post-operation physical status. The question to be asked here is whether present day health care systems are structured and staffed in such a way that the psychosocial and behavioural factors involved are timely detected, adequately treated and wherever possible prevented from (re)occurring. A related question is whether there are methods and approaches available to assess, treat and prevent such problems or disorders. Even if one has to conclude that particular knowledge and skills are not sufficiently used, one still cannot simply go on to state that there is therefore a problem. The only justification for such an assertion could be that there is a clear demand and need for that particular knowledge that thus far has not adequately been met.

The aims of the present article are to point out that international and national health and health-related policies all around the globe demand a massive influx of psychosocial and behavioural knowledge and skills in the care and promotion of health in order to be successful. In order to make that knowledge and skills accessible to health care policy makers, health care professionals, and the public, national and international programmes should be developed aimed at completing and partially replacing the currently prevailing biomedical orientation in health and health care by a psychosocial and behavioural approach.

2. HEALTH FOR ALL

Just ten years ago, in 1977, WHO's policy-making body, the World Health Assembly, made a momentous decision. It decided that the main social targets of governments and WHO in the coming decades should be the attainment by all people of the world by the year 2000 of a level of health that will permit them to lead a socially and economically productive life. This is popularly known as Health for All by the Year 2000 or HFA/2000, (WHO, 1981).

What does the policy mean for people throughout the world and what relevance does behavioural science knowledge and skills have for its implementation and success?

If we try to sum up the essence of HFA/2000 the following picture emerges. People including health personnel and their elected representatives should work together to promote health, prevent disease, alleviate unavoidable disease and disability, improve the process of being born and growing up, insure that all are healthy enough to work productively and to participate in the social life of the community, and finally, facilitate growing old gracefully and dying in dignity.

The underlying assumption in all these aspects of HFA/2000 is that there is a very intimate relationship between people's behaviour, their lifestyles, and their level of health. The impact of behaviour on the burden of illness and mortality is reflected in the fact that nonadherence to hygiene and safety prescriptions, alcohol and drug abuse, smoking, nonadherence to proven medical regimens, bad eating and lack of skills for coping with stress are disproportionately present among persons suffering from ill health or dying premature deaths, that is, before the usual life expectancy (Hamburg *et al.*, 1982). Each year millions of deaths all over the world are caused by infectious disease, accidents and violence including homicide and suicide, and diseases such as cardiovascular disease, cancers, diabetes, cirrhosis of the liver and respiratory diseases which often have developed as a result of careless, dangerous or unhealthy behaviour. Many of these leading causes of death are chronic and progressively disabling diseases, which means that years of limitation in function and associated health care costs may precede death.

Among the almost 500 million people living in the United States and the countries of the European Economic Community, an estimated 70 million have cancer. Each year at least 150 million people are injured by accidents, poisoning or violence serious enough to require medical attention or to restrict activity for a considerable period of time. As much as 15% of the population experience a mental disorder of a more or less severe degree.

Much of the disease and disability that the people in industrialized countries have is caused by overeating, overdrinking, overdriving cars, overdriving themselves, overdrugging themselves, overpolluting the air, overpolluting the water and over-sedentary living in towns.

In developing countries main causes of illness are malnutrition (including energy malnutrition and vitamin A deficiency blindness), malaria, acute respiratory infections, diarrhoea, leprosy, tuberculosis and common infectious diseases of childhood. Many of these illnesses are contracted, or one could even say, caused by behaviour of people.

The question then arises, what answers are there to such diverse problems as these? They obviously cannot be dealt with adequately by a classical medical care model, that is, by waiting for people to become ill and then treating them or nursing them until the acute episode of the illness passes, or taking it for granted that people will become chronically ill and providing them with medical care for the rest of their lives.

2.1 Towards a New Model of Health Care

Is it at all possible, one could ask, to identify a universal model that could be adapted to different circumstances? An international conference, held in Alma Ata in 1978 declared that Health for All could be attained through health systems based on what is called primary health care. What could systems like these look like in different countries, taking into account the type of health problems that have been described above? According to the statement that was formulated in the Alma Ata declaration, health systems based on primary health care or with an emphasis on primary health care have the following characteristics (WHO, 1978). First of all, they reflect the social, economic and political characteristics of the country, state or community in question. Secondly, they give priority to those most in need. Furthermore, they address the main health problems in the community. Fourth they provide promotive, preventive, curative and rehabilitative services. They involve other related sectors such as agriculture and animal husbandry, food, industry and most importantly, education.

Health systems with an emphasis on primary health care also rely on maximum community and individual self-reliance in planning, operation and control. They make full use of local resources and ensure country-wide coverage of defined health programmes. They use health technology that is appropriate—an implication essential for the role of psychology to play in primary health care—that wherever possible social and behavioural alternatives for medical and technical measures should be used as widely as possible. Such health systems are sustained by a supportive referral system and health care is provided by health teams in which traditional medical, social, psychosocial and behavioural expertise are brought together.

The Declaration of Alma Ata also defined a number of essential elements that primary health care should include: there are eight of these essential elements but within the framework of this article, the first one is the most essential, namely: "Primary health care includes: education concerning prevailing health problems and methods of preventing and controlling them." This element, which in abbreviated form can be labelled health promotion or promotion of lifestyles or behaviour patterns that are conducive to good health, really is the antithesis of the classical medical care model and it is one of the main pillars of a health system based on primary health care.

2.2 Promotion of Health

What does health promotion imply? It is an evolving concept. Some of the main components of health promotion at this time are:

—fostering healthy lifestyles:

—fostering social, economic and environmental conditions conducive to health:

—trying to attain these two by raising awareness about health matters in individuals and communities:

—by enabling people to cope with their and their family's health problems both general and mental health problems; and

—by encouraging social support or the use of social support.

Further, health promotion implies judicious taxation that promotes health. It also implies producing and consuming food and drink conducive to health. It emphasizes adequate and appropriate exercise. It emphasizes teaching people to use adequate and healthy sleeping patterns. It emphasizes that people are educated and work in conformity with their physical and mental capacity. It emphasizes suitable living arrangements in terms of housing and social support within reach. It emphasizes the improvement of the physical, psychological and social environment of people.

2.3 Health-Damaging Lifestyles

There exists enough scientific evidence on the effects of certain types of behaviour to classify them as well-established and unambiguous forms of risk behaviour, such as excessive smoking, alcohol use in excess, misuse of medical and mood-altering drugs, inadequate eating patterns, lack of physical exercise, dangerous driving, violent behaviour and inadequate or deficient stress management skills. The negative health effects of these behaviours are in fact so well studied and—at least in principle—generally agreed upon that both large-scale intervention programmes and primary health care individually-oriented programmes are called for which aim at reducing their occurrence. Several recent WHO documents explicitly state that the psychological sciences have to make a significant contribution here, such as:

—analysis of the subjective meaning and of the functions which these forms of behaviour serve for the individual or social group (e.g. youth cultures) concerned;

—identification of the social forces which tend (directly or indirectly) to stabilize and encourage these forms of risk behaviour;

—development, testing and comparison of different intervention strategies aimed both at the risk-taking individuals and at the social forces which favour such risk-taking;

—assistance in the provision of these interventions on all levels of care, in particular, primary health care;
—evaluation of all intervention programmes.

A reduction in the occurrence of such risk behaviours would certainly lead to an improvement of the health status in a general population—and this is why much of WHO's programme on Health for All by the Year 2000 focuses on changing these well-established and highly relevant forms of risk behaviours.

2.4 Other Types of Risk Behaviour

The forms of risk behaviour just mentioned explain only a part of the variance of behaviour-related health outcomes. Both research and programmes of health education and disease intervention tend to concentrate on these forms, probably because only individuals seem to be involved and because attempts to reduce the health risks can be addressed at individuals rather than at social institutions or persons in authority. As a result, the concept of risk behaviour is in danger of being narrowed down to "misbehaviour", like excessive smoking and alcohol drinking. There are other forms of suspected risk behaviour, but presently available knowledge and general acceptance is perhaps not sufficient to start intervention programmes. The available knowledge in psychology though is sufficient to justify major efforts directed at suspected health damage by some widespread and socially-accepted lifestyles. Among these are (see e.g. Hammonds and Scheirer, 1984):

—patterns of behaviour prevailing in the occupational world (chronic stress resulting from excessive time pressure and structural social conflicts in the working situation; overambition; alcoholism; shift work; social modularization of unemployed persons, underemployment);
—chronic stress resulting from gender-specific role expectations (e.g. double strain on women in familial and occupational roles; inferior social status of women and girls in many countries; chronic suppression of emotions in male role expectation);
—overdemands on individual or family capacities to adapt to rapid social change (urbanization, modernization, secularization, computerization, increasing demands on occupational and local mobility).
—risk behaviour reduced by the health care system itself "medicalization" of every-day life; patient role as passive recipient of medical treatment; impersonalization and emphasis on technological aspects of health and health care.

2.5 Health-Enhancing Lifestyles

Enhancing lifestyles that are health promoting, maintaining or improving the health status of individuals and the population in general is clearly an important aspect of the HFA/2000 strategy. Unfortunately, the concept of positive health is presently neither clearly defined nor well-studied empirically. If the very promising approach of supporting a healthy lifestyle is to be pursued, there is an urgent need for a much greater influence of psychological knowledge in studies and programmes directed towards establishing the positive health effects of lifestyles or elements of lifestyles. It is of special importance that within this frame of reference the focus should be on healthy people and identification of those elements in their behaviour and resources that make them distinguishable from the less healthy. Research findings so far (Steptoe and Mathews, 1984) point to several aspects of lifestyles which probably contribute to maintenance of good health:

—sufficient income plus adequate command of the work and domestic situation;

—adequate psychological and behavioural mechanisms for coping with emerging problems;

—social integration and sufficient social support in times of crisis;

—self-esteem and feelings of sufficient internal control over one's life;

—beliefs which emphasize personal influence on health and well-being.

2.6 Induction of Changes of Lifestyle

Inherent in the lifestyle approach and therefore inherent in the primary health care emphasis within HFA/2000, the intention is to introduce change in prevailing lifestyles: to spread health-enhancing, and to reduce health-damaging lifestyles. From a behavioural science point of view, the attempt to introduce a healthy lifestyle as a normal way of life to society poses some general problems which have consequences for the content and the provision of care. For a balance has to be found between a legitimate intent to influence other people's way of life to their own benefit on the one hand, and the basic right of these same people to choose their own way of life and define for themselves what is beneficial on the other hand. This balance can obviously be established only if the "objects" of the intervention have an equal say in the planning and realization of the intervention programme.

The methodologies for such a participative approach are at present unsatisfactory, need further development and will be dependent upon a massive influence of behavioural science knowledge both in terms of research and in terms of the development and provision of health care. Furthermore, if intervention programmes focus exclusively on the well established forms of risk behaviour (like excessive smoking, alcohol abuse, overeating, etc.) they can easily lead to moralistic attitudes (e.g. victim blaming) and this imposes an additional burden on individuals already at increased risk. In order to avoid these attitudes, health care planners have to turn to psychologists for help in developing a concept which can reconcile personal responsibility for, and external influences on, individual risk behaviour and resulting health effects.

Finally, promoting healthy lifestyles as a normal way of life has to safeguard against a danger of "healthism": establishing an ideal of a healthy socially fully integrated psychologically well-balanced individual as a social norm. Before and after the year 2000 physical and emotional suffering, loneliness, poverty and misery, illness and dying will remain part of the human condition: if the ideal healthy person were established as a norm, this could on the one hand help many people to adopt health-enhancing lifestyles; this very norm, however, would on the other hand, push all those persons who do not correspond to this norm to the margins of normal society.

Inasmuch as developing the ideally healthy lifestyle is dependent upon the socio-economic position and "richness" of a person, such a development would only lead to an increase in social inequity in health and social influence. It has to be pointed out that at present the focus of the health promotion movement is on health but very little is known about the effects which cognitive changes have on actual behaviour. One of the reasons for this present state of affairs is that behavioural science knowledge and skills have only been used in the area of health education and health promotion to a very limited extent.

Another area of neglect thus far has been the development of individual health promotion in the form of counseling individuals who start their career as a patient in the health care system on how to change their lifestyle and develop more healthy styles of life. Behavioural counseling in primary health care is still in its infant stage (Carnwath and Miller, 1986). One of the implications of HFA/2000 however is that at all levels of care, but in particular in primary health care, and in all health promotion programmes, the application of behavioural methods of change and improving health should be fostered. The apparent success of certain health promoting groups such as Alcoholics Anonymous and Weight Watchers, Coronary Group, self-help groups and other mutual aid groups, point to the fact that relatively stable changes in health behaviour are favoured by factors which for a long time have already been disclosed by psychological research, especially within the framework of learning theories such as success modeling, social reinforcement integration into every.day life and participation in the planning and the carrying out of activities. The introduction of these and other factors in health care delivery should be extended, tested and evaluated.

This points to the importance of social support as well as the importance of individuals' use of skills to mobilize social networks and to make use of social relationships in times of crisis (Mechanic, 1983). The individual's capacity to mobilize social networks signals the importance of what in present day behavioural science is called the coping repertoire or the coping styles of individuals and of groups.

Since chronic conflict and stress have to be considered as major factors influencing behaviour-related health outcomes, adequate coping capacities of individuals are obviously an important element of health-enhancing lifestyles. The current state of scientific knowledge in psychology indicates that there is sufficient evidence, for example based on studies of coping with chronic disease such as cancer, to prove the relevance of the concept. However, many questions need decisive answers. For example: in what way does coping capacity depend on a material base which people dispose of? Or, can general coping strategies be identified which are particularly promising in various issues of conflict resolution, problem solving, decision making and stress reduction? Active confrontation and fighting spirit versus passive resignation and denial or avoidance provide examples of vastly different coping styles which may lead to many different health outcomes. What are the criteria to distinguish more or less *successful* coping strategies? Or, what makes one person a better coper than another? Or are coping strategies simply patterns of social behaviour which are accessible to induced change? Or, are there differences in the social distribution of successful coping strategies, for example, based on education, social strata, gender, religion, age, etc?

A general conclusion from the above and an element of HFA/2000 therefore is that if individual or group behaviour as well as the social conditions that influence it are to be regarded as basic factors contributing to the genesis of health and illness then obviously psychological and behavioural factors have to be included in the planning and provision of health care, and in finding ways of improving and promoting health.

The traditional biomedical approach to health has thus to be extended and complemented by the psychosocial and behavioural approach. Although there is some awareness of this necessity in most countries, both knowledge and application of psychosocial and behavioural strategies and techniques in health care and in particular in primary health care are still relatively scarce.

2.7 The Psychosocial and Behavioural Component of Primary Health Care (PHC)

With the foregoing in mind we now are able to define with more precision the psychosocial and behavioural component of health care and therewith the role of behavioural sciences within health systems based on the PHC philosophy.

The psychosocial and behavioural component of health care comprises the following quite distinct, but unfortunately often confused, areas:

The first area emphasizes the practical relevance of psychological or behavioural science skills in general health care. These skills are of vital importance in e.g.:

—improving the functioning of general health services;

—supporting overall socio-economic development;

—enhancing the quality of life;

—promoting mental and emotional health as positive life goals.

These have seldom formed part of the tasks actually assigned to health care workers. They are essential PHC skills.

The secondary area concerns:

—the diagnosis and treatment (including rehabilitation) of mentally and neurologically ill persons;

—the prevention of mental and neurological disorders.

These aspects can be partially the responsibility of primary health care workers, but often also require the involvement of specialists.

2.8 On Appropriate Care

One of the most evident implications of the psychosocial and behavioural component in the Health for All strategy is the introduction of psychosocial and behavioural analysis and intervention as part of the activity of primary health care workers. This requires a massive influx of skills and knowledge from scientific and professional psychology.

But how is this going to happen? It is apparent that in most other countries much greater emphasis is given to physical than to psychosocial and mental health problems in both training and practice of those involved in primary health care. The most cursory examination of primary health care manuals and textbooks makes this apparent. This stands in clear contrast to the widely accepted and acknowledged fact that psychosocial and mental health problems are widely prevalent, constituting a distressing burden in the population, are very often brought to the attention of primary care practitioners, are often not identified, and are very frequently inadequately assessed and treated. This statement holds true for most states and communities despite considerable differences in the organization and delivery of primary health care.

In some countries the vast majority of doctors in primary health care work single-handedly, whereas in others the majority of general practitioners collaborate in partnership (i.e. groups of doctors cooperating together) or interdisciplinary teams, usually comprised of social workers and nurses. In other countries such as the United States, patients may have a family physician but are also able to directly call on specialists such as pediatricians or gynacologists who have a specific responsibility for the category of patients within their area of expertise.

Research suggests that in countries where primary health care depends on physicians, such as is the case in most parts of the world, these practitioners as a group presently lack interest and expertise to respond to psychological and mental health problems of their patients. There would appear to be two main avenues open to improvement of this unsatisfactory situation, each of which carries profound organizational, practical and research implications. These are:

(a) The primary health care worker is guided and trained to reorient his or her way of dealing with help seekers in such a way as to include psychosocial or behavioural mental health care in his or her practice. This necessarily implicates a need for improvement in knowledge and skills to ensure that necessary tasks can be carried out economically and effectively; it also implies that psychological techniques for widespread dissemination—techniques that are simple and easily applicable—are developed and tested. Understandably in developing, and much less understandably in developed countries, health care training has to this point heavily emphasized the physical or somatic aspects of diseases and of health.

Little instruction is usually given on the importance of psychological or social factors in the development of physical disorders or more purely psychological problems often encountered in practice. It is also striking how little attention is given to psychological and behavioural aspects of health in the content of examinations and in the evaluation of courses in the curricula of all different kinds of health workers. Consequently, health care practitioners do not perceive themselves as and are not by consequence the right people to deal with these problems. When faced with them, they usually feel inadequate and may respond with lack of sympathy or inappropriate competent advice.

It is common for a primary health care physician to say to a mother with a seriously disabled child "there's nothing wrong with your child", when what is meant is that the physician can detect no physical abnormality or sign of physical disease and suspects that the symptoms have a psychological cause. Following this first avenue, comprehensive primary health care as meant by the Alma Ata Declaration and as meant in the WHO programme of Health for All by the Year 2000 can only be realized if a considerable reorientation in basic and additional training of doctors, nurses and other primary health care workers is effected.

(b) The second avenue is essentially based on the viewpoint that it is impossible for a primary health care worker to combine in one and the same person the necessary and sufficient knowledge and skills for dealing with both the physical and psychological or mental health complaints or problems of patients.

The logical consequence of this point of view is that on the primary health care level, direct access and availability of both generalists in physical health care and in psychological health care, should be present. This in turn implies that primary health care should be carried out by a combination of different disciplines of which behavioural sciences or psychology is one. The suggestion here is that psychologists as practitioners have an important role to play in primary health care, a viewpoint that has been advocated for more than a decade (Broadhurst, 1972).

Indeed, in a number of countries in Europe, for example, England and the Netherlands, it is estimated that one in 5–7 psychologists are already working with general practitioners. In countries in other parts of the world such as Cuba and Argentina psychologists are also clearly present at the PHC level. The rationale behind this approach is that primary care practitioners are much more likely to identify psychological and mental health disorders in their patients and to use mental health or psychological specialists for treatment, consultation and referral, when general health and mental health services are brought together through integrated attachment schemes or linkage models within or on the primary health care level. Some authors have even drawn the conclusion that unless a major portion of the psychological service in primary care settings is provided by professionals like psychologists, a gap will remain between patient needs for mental health service and minimal physician's response (Wright and Burns, 1986). Such a condition is not in the public interest. Primary mental health psychology and primary mental health psychologists therefore should be seen as an essential element of primary health care.

When one asks the question: Which of the two avenues described here is generally

Table 1 Categories of psychological problems amenable to primary psychological intervention (Adapted from Kincey, 1974)

Category	*Description*
(a) Problems of anxiety and stress	Generalized anxiety, panic attacks, phobias, obsessional ideas or rituals, stress-induced or aggravated illnesses, e.g. migraine, asthma, cardiovascular disease.
(b) Habit disorders	Various habitual behaviours that led to personal distress, ill-health or social problems, e.g. smoking, obesity, bulimia, problem drinking, enuresis, encopresis, drug addiction.
(c) Educational, occupational difficulties or decisions	Choice of transition points throughout life span, e.g. leaving school, change of job, retirement. Problems that arise in the educational–occupational context, e.g. study problems, lack of confidence and social skills.
(d) Interpersonal-social-marital problems	Problems arising out of relationships with others, e.g. shyness, unassertiveness, marital discord, psychosexual problems, antisocial and aggressive behaviour.
(e) Psychological adjustment to physical illness and other significant life events	Adjustment to psychological trauma of illness and hospitalization. Adjustment to chronic disability. Childbirth, accident, terminal illness, death.

to be preferred?, the answer can only be that this is not the right question to ask. First of all, not enough research has been done thus far to allow a clear choice between both alternatives. And secondly, the choice between both avenues depends, among other things, on the cultural, social and financial situation that is present in a specific community or state. Furthermore, it might well be and very probably is the case, that both approaches are not as contradictory or mutually exclusive as they seem at first glance. The second approach requires well-designed studies in order to explore and differentiate the health role of psychologists in primary care from that of primary care physicians, nurses and social workers. It might very well turn out that the particular contributions that a psychologist could make in primary health care and to each primary medicine speciality are different in different communities and (sub) cultures. Dependent on such factors, psychologists' role may vary from an independent helper in the primary health care level to providing only support and knowledge to and sharing skills with other primary health care practitioners.

2.9 Problems Amenable to Psychosocial and Behavioural Interventions in Primary Health Care

An important question to be asked is: What kind of problems are amenable to psychological interventions in primary health care? In a survey of general practitioners in the United Kingdom the most common problems deemed particularly suitable by a sample of GPs for such interventions were (in order): phobias, chronic anxiety, obsessional disorders, smoking problems, drinking problems, psychosexual problems and interpersonal problems (Marzillier and Hall, 1987).

According to the present author the answer to the question: What sort of problems would be most effectively dealt with by psychological knowledge and skills in primary health care? can be answered by referring to the categories of problem areas that Kincey (1974) has described, and that are shown in *Table 1*.

CONCLUSION

The application of relevant knowledge to psychosocial and behavioural factors and interventions related to health will result in a better and more rational provision of services and care as well as in an increase of self responsibility for their health status among people.

In order to introduce such knowledge and skills in health care in an appropriate degree, national, regional, and local policies should be developed. The World Health Organization's programme for psychological and social factors in health continues to address these problems. For additional information contact the author.

References

Broadhurst, A. (1972). Clinical psychology and the general practitioner. *British Medical Journal,* **1**, 793–795.

Carnwath, T. and Miller, D. (1986). *Behavioural psychotherapy in primary care: a practice manual.* London: Academic Press.

Diekstra, R. F. W. (1989). *Psychosocial and behavioural aspects of health and development.* Geneva: World Health Organisation.

Hamburg, D. A., Elliott, G. R. and Parson, D. L. (Eds.) (1982). *Health and behavior: frontiers of research in the biobehavioral sciences.* Washington: National Academy Press.
Hammonds, B. L. and Scheirer, C. J. (Eds.) (1984). *Psychology and health. The master lecturer series.* Washington: American Psychological Association.
Kincey, J. A. (1974). General practice and clinical psychology—some arguments for a closer liason. *Journal of the Royal College of General Practitioners,* **24**, 882–888.
Lipowski, Z. Y. (1988) Somatization: the concept and its clinical application. *American Journal of Psychiatry,* **145,** 11, 1350–1378.
Marzillier, J. S. and Hall, J. (1987). *What is clinical psychology?* Oxford: Oxford University Press.
Mechanic, D. (Ed.) (1983). *Handbook of health, health care and the professions.* New York: Free Press.
Steptoe, A. and Mathews, A. (Eds.) (1984). *Health care and human behaviour.* London: Academic Press.
World Health Organisation (1978). *Primary health care: alma ata.* Geneva: World Health Organisation.
World Health Organisation (1981). Global strategy for health for all by the year 2000. Geneva: World Health Organisation.
Wright, L. and Burns, B. J. (1986). Primary mental health care: A "find" for psychology? *Professional Psychology: Research and Practice,* **17**, 6, 560–564.

CHAPTER 3

HEALTH PSYCHOLOGY WITHIN THE EUROPEAN HEALTH CARE SYSTEMS

L.R. SCHMIDT and G.E. DLUGOSCH

Fachbereich I – Psychologie, Universität Trier
Postfach 3825, 5500 Trier, Germany

This paper attempts to describe the current status of health psychology, particularly involving primary prevention work, within the diverse health care systems in Europe. Considerable problems were experienced in obtaining comprehensive data from all countries and it was difficult to establish the reliability and validity of the data which was obtained. The major part of the paper describes the health care systems and place of health psychology in Finland, Germany, Spain, Sweden and the United Kingdom. Although there are a few impressive developments in primary prevention and health education, the overall picture of this work is not very encouraging. However, there are some promising developments with the formation of new societies, journals and postgraduate programs. Health psychology needs to define appropriate outcome criteria for evaluating preventive initiatives and must take account of ethical and social issues in pursuing health related behaviour change. In Europe, as in many other countries, psychologists need to define and promote their potential contribution to primary prevention and it may well be that changes must take place in health care systems before these contributions can be fully realised.

1. INTRODUCTORY REMARKS

Analyzing the state of health psychology in Europe can be regarded a challenging task. Although the definition of *health psychology* by Matarazzo (1980) has been widely accepted, there is still considerable debate about its contents, goals and applications (cf., Schmidt, Schwenkmezger & Dlugosch, 1990). While issues of secondary and tertiary prevention in the medical field are increasingly provided by the disciplines of medical psychology or behavioral medicine, "true" health psychology, involving primary prevention in the health and medical field, is still quite rare in many European countries. However, most governments and other official institutions claim health as an extremely important goal for the whole country and participate in activities like the global WHO strategy "Health for all by the year 2000" (cf., WHO, 1987).

Except for a few outstanding research projects and practical models (some of them are described below), primary prevention is still not being supported adequately. One possible explanation for this situation might be found in the power struggle of different professions competing in the health field. Forgács and Kökény (1989) elucidate this statement in their review of the Long-term National Programme of Health Promotion started in 1987 by the Hungarian government by concluding that "... the efforts to convince doctors of the importance of the programme failed because doctors consider it to be the rival resources to be devoted to curative care." (p. 55).

2. COMPARING EUROPEAN HEALTH CARE SYSTEMS

Unfortunately, there is a lack of background information about the structure of the different health systems, their political and economic conditions, sufficient epidemiological data of each country and the nature of the data sources. In order to discuss the situation of health psychology in Europe thoroughly, we need comparable indicators of health and health systems as well as several kinds of criteria (cf., Alber, 1988, 1989; Buchholz, 1988; Deppe, 1983; Deppe & Lenhardt, 1990; Gäfgen, 1986; Koch et al., 1986; Maynard, 1982; Schach, 1985; U. Schmidt, 1983; Schneider, 1990; Schwefel, 1987). However, at this point in time the only sound data base seems to exist for the OECD countries (Alber, 1988; OECD, 1990).

In Table 1, *potential indicators of health and health care systems* are listed. Such indicators can provide a scientific basis for a characterization of the specific health systems and for evaluative comparisons between countries.

Table 1 Indicators of health care systems and indicators of health

Indicators of health care systems
- broader sections of the health system political system; public health; environmental policies; social services; training and education of health professionals
- formal structure of the health system steering; legal regulations; financial regulations; insurance policies (agencies, coverage) organisation and administration of in-patient and out-patient services; freedom of choice regarding diagnosis and treatment distribution of curative and preventive services (regional balance; number of professionals; number of hospital beds; federal and private health care organisations and institutions; paraprofessional and lay participation)
- efficiency of the health system costs; cost-effectiveness; supply – demand
Indicators of health
- epidemiological data life expectancy; infant mortality rate; morbidity; mortality; causes of death and premature death (incl. accidents, homicide, and suicide)
- health status (vs. health risks) individual (physical, psychological) social (family, subpopulations, community, society) environmental (pollution, wastes, safety, housing) political (employment, national and international politics, wars)
- immunogens vs. pathogens
- health behavior (vs. risk behavior) individual (exercise, nutrition, stress management, family planning, etc.) environmental political (supporting primary prevention projects like drug or smoking prevention; health education, health promotion, public health activities)

Table 2 A typology of health systems (adapted from Field, 1989b)

Health System	*Type 1* *Emergent*	*Type 2* *Pluralistic*	*Type 3* *Insurance/ Social Security*	*Type 4* *National Health Service*	*Type 5* *Socialized*
General Definition	Health care as item of personal consumption	Health care as consumer good or service	Health care as insured/guaranteed consumer good or service	Health care as state supported consumer good or service	Health care as state provided public service
Position of the Physician	Solo entrepreneur	Solo entrepreneur and member of variety of groups/ organizations	Solo entrepreneur and member of medical organizations	Solo entrepreneur and member of medical organizations	State employee and member of medical organizations
Role of Professional Associations	Powerful	Very strong	Strong	Fairly strong	Weak or non-existent
Ownership of Facilities	Private	Private and public	Private and public	Mostly public	Entirely public
Economic Transfers	Direct	Direct and Indirect	Mostly Indirect	Indirect	Entirely Indirect
Prototypes	USA	USA ; Switzerland South Africa	Sweden; France; Germany; Japan Canada; Italy	Great Britain; Australia	Soviet Russia Eastern Europe; Cuba

Table 3 Selected indicators and rank order of OECD countries (adapted from Alber, 1988). Note that the data stem from 1982; meanwhile several changes took place and especially the expenditures of the countries are much higher. A more recent analysis was published shortly after the submission of this paper (cf., OECD, 1990).

Country	*Health expenditure (% GNP)*		*% Public share a)*		*Infant mortality rate at 40*		*Life expectancy female at 40*		*Life expectancy male b)*		*Employ-ment rate c)*		*Number of physicians c)*		*Number of beds*		*Hospital admissions (per year) (days)*		*Length of hospital stay*	
Belgium	6.2	12	92	1.5	11.7	12	37.5	14	32.0	12.5	4.5	8.5	27	3	95	8	13.9	7	14	5
Denmark	6.8	8	84	4.5	8.2	5	39.2	9	33.9	6	4.8	7	24	5	74	11	19.2	2.5	12	2.5
Finland	6.6	9.5	79	7.5	6.0	1	39.0	10	31.8	14	5.9	3	22	8	156	1	20.9	1	22	10
France	9.3	3	71	11.5	9.3	7	40.2	5	33.2	9	4.5	8.5	22	8	116	5	11.8	10.5	14	5
FRG	8.2	5	81	6	10.9	9	38.6	11	32.9	10	2.2	14	24	5	111	7	18.1	4	19	8.5
Italy	7.2	7	84	4.5	13.0	13	39.5	8	33.7	7	2.6	12	32	1	77	10	15.4	6	12	2.5
NL	8.7	4	79	7.5	8.3	6	40.7	2	34.7	4	7.1	2	21	10	120	4	11.8	10.5	34	13
Portugal	5.7	14	71	11.5	20.2	14	38.0	13	32.0	12.5	2.4	13	22	8	51	14	9.6	12	14	5
Spain	6.3	11	72	10	9.6	8	39.6	7	34.5	5	3.0	10	28	2	54	13	9.2	13	15	7
Sweden	9.7	2	92	1.5	6.8	3	40.4	4	34.9	3	7.8	1	24	5	140	2	19.2	2.5	23	11
Switzerl.	7.8	6	65	13	8.0	4	40.7	2	35.1	2	5.6	4	16	12	115	6	12.8	8	25	12
UK	5.9	13	88	3	11.0	10	38.2	12	32.7	11	5.2	6	13	14	81	9	12.7	9	19	8.5
USA	10.6	1	42	14	11.2	11	39.8	6	33.3	8	5.3	5	19	11	59	12	17.0	5	10	1
Japan	6.6	9.5	74	9	6.6	2	40.7	2	35.9	1	2.9	11	14	13	121	3	6.7	14	55	14

a) death rates of children up to 1 year per 1.000 live births
b) within the health system
c) per 10.000 inhabitants

Table 2 introduces a *typology of health systems* based on Field (1989a, b).

Table 3 contains some *basic indicators* of different European health systems. It reflects the disparities between these countries as well as the comparison with the USA and Japan.

Issues of the overall approach and the functioning of a health system are, of course, important points of continuing discussion. Comparing the health systems of France, FRG and Great Britain, Alber (1989) claims that systems controlled by the state are more adaptive than private systems of medical care.

3. GOALS AND OBJECTIVES OF THE INQUIRY

The present comparison mainly focuses on the area of *primary prevention*, represented by health promotion, health education, public health and primary health care (Diekstra & Jansen, 1990; Harris, 1980; Winett et al., 1989).

Our analysis was based on two information sources:

1) an analysis of existing English and German literature (see reference list)

2) a letter (dated February 13, 1990) from us to the health departments of every European country, international organizations (WHO, EC, IUHE) and some colleagues and recommended specialists in the field to find out about the state of the art of the health systems in general and health psychology in particular.

The responses were quite disappointing: Out of 29 European countries contacted, only 12 replied (namely: Belgium, Denmark, FRG, GDR, Hungary, Italy, Luxemburg, Monaco, Netherlands, Northern Ireland, Sweden and Switzerland).

Unfortunately, even the comparative literature provided by international organizations was found to contain some methodological problems (e.g., WHO, 1989; International Union for Health Education [IUHE], 1988). The publications of a few specialists regarding health and health care systems seemed more valid (Alber, 1988, 1989; Deppe, 1983; Deppe & Lenhardt, 1990; Field, 1989a, b; Keil et al., 1990 with regard to Finland, FRG, Sweden and UK; Tietze, 1989).

4. DESCRIPTION OF SELECTED EUROPEAN HEALTH SYSTEMS WITH SPECIAL REGARD TO THE STATE OF HEALTH PSYCHOLOGY

In the following we will sketch the role of health psychology within the health systems of the selected countries (in alphabetical order): Finland, Germany (Federal Republic of Germany and former German Democratic Republic), Spain, Sweden, and United Kingdom.

Although the selection was extremely limited, a certain representativity of the different kinds of health systems was aimed at (cf., Alber, 1988; Field, 1989b). Furthermore, our decision was influenced by the quality and the quantity of the materials we received and the literature we gathered.

In general the most organized and developed area of health psychology in Europe is the field of *health education*. An International Union for Health Education (IUHE) and several national health education centres or committees exist. Every few years a comparison of the current state of health education in the various European countries is being published by the International Union for Health

Education. Our description is mainly based on their latest edition from 1988. Even though the same term, "health education", is used, its meaning and organisation varies greatly within the different European countries. Being a part of the health system, health education depends for example on such criteria as the level of centralization or the funding by governmental agencies vs. private organisations. We decided to include health education and health promotion as areas of concern for health psychology although in practice psychologists have rarely been given a proper opportunity to play an important role in contributing to the goals of health maintenance and disease prevention. In fact, in many European countries there were no health psychologists employed by the health system at the present time.

4.1 FINLAND

Health system

We do not want to go into details about the Finnish health system since its characteristics are very similar to the Swedish system described below. We decided to include it anyhow because the areas of health promotion and health education seem to be quite well developed. These efforts might be at least partially due to the fact that in the statistics of the early 1970's Finland had a low ranking with respect to various health indicators.

Health psychology

Good examples of *health promotion* are found in the national surveys of health behaviour as described by Kalimo (1988):

> "Since the early 1960s nationwide surveys have been conducted in Finland to provide information about essential issues of health, health care and health promotion in order to develop the national health policy and the measures following from it . . . Another characteristic of the studies has been the close relationship between the national health and/or social security administration and the research activities. The studies have been action-oriented and the decision-makers have been involved in setting the objectives of the study as well as in the application of the results to health and social security policy making and related planning and administration in the Ministry of Social Affairs and Health, the Social Insurance Institution, as well as other relevant institutions." (p. 134).

The following nationwide studies are mentioned:

- National Health and Social Security Interview Surveys, conducted by the Research Institute for Social Security of the Social Insurance Institution, Finland, in collaboration with the National Board of Health, in 1964, 1968, and 1976
- Mini-Finland Health Survey, conducted by the Rehabilitation Research Centre and the Research Institute for Social Security of the Social Insurance Institution, Finland, in 1977–1980
- Nationwide Questionnaire Survey of Sickness Absenteeism from Work, conducted by the Research Institute for Social Security of the Social Insurance Institution, Finland, in 1974
- National Questionnaire Surveys of Health Behaviour, conducted by the Public Health Institute annually since 1978
- National Interview Surveys of Health Education, conducted by the National Board of Health twice annually since 1979
- National Questionnaire Surveys of Occupational Health Care, conducted by the Research Institute for Social Security of the Social Insurance Institution, Finland, in 1981 and 1985

The goal of the Juvenile Health Habit Study 1977–1985 (cf., Rimpelä, Rimpelä, Rahkonen & Teperi, 1988) was to develop a nationwide information system to follow up changes in health behaviour in young people. Key areas were the process of maturation, human relations and social support mechanisms, and perceived health, symptoms and disease episodes.

Other on-going projects described by Juusela (1988) include studies on smoking in children and young people; smoking habits of the adult population; research on the cessation of tobacco smoking; studies of the economic consequences of smoking; other than tobacco studies; and general health education programmes.

The North Karelia Project is an outstanding example of community-based prevention of cardiovascular disease. Due to the extremely high prevalence of cardiovascular diseases in Finland, this project was started in 1972. Strategies such as information provision, persuasion, training, social support, environmental change and community organization have been implemented (cf., Puska, 1984). The outcome data seem to be promising but follow-up data are still being gathered and analyzed.

4.2 GERMANY

4.2.1 FEDERAL REPUBLIC OF GERMANY

Health system

The structure of the German health system is very complicated (for detailed overviews see Buchholz, 1988; Gäfgen & Lampert, 1982; Keil et al., 1990; WHO, 1989). It is represented by the public sector, the outpatient medical service (primary health care), the outpatient non-medical service (nurses, psychologists), inpatient medical service (hospital), rehabilitation clinics and drug supply (cf., Buchholz, 1988). The relationships within and between these sectors are extremely complex. For example, the outpatient medical service not only depends on the patient, the physician and the health insurance coverage but also on the rules and regulations of the "Kassenärztliche Vereinigung", a representative body of the physicians who as a whole are responsible for outpatient services for certain defined areas.

The National Institute of Health ("Bundesgesundheitsamt") is an independent federal institution with 7 subdivisons, employing 1800 people altogether.

After the USA, the German health system is the second most expensive at present. Schäfer and Wachtel (1989) estimate the annual health care costs to be 240.000.000.000 DM. In sharp contrast to this very high level of expenditure is the lack of sound information as to what this money is being spent on as well as an only average ranking with regard to health indicators (cf., Bundesgesundheitsamt, 1989).

According to Deppe and Lenhardt (1990), special characteristics of the West German health system are:

—low employment rate of personnel in the medical field other than physicians, especially for nurses;
—extremely high incomes for physicians;
—public social health insurance, covering the costs of mainly private health services especially provided by physicians in private practice and drug companies.

Following Deppe (1983), it also seems to be unique for Germany to strictly separate inpatient and outpatient medical care.

Health psychology

Surprisingly enough, in the FRG "true" health psychology does not have more manpower than in other European countries where a lot less money is being spent within the health sector. This might partially be due to the dominance of the medical profession in the health system and the lack of interdisciplinary primary health care centers. The German Minister for Youth, Family, Women, and Health (Bundesminister für Jugend, Familie, Frauen und Gesundheit, 1988) mentions, that 923.440 professionals are employed within the health system. This figure does not include one single psychologist. Obviously, psychologists working in the health system in Germany are not recognized officially.

As in many other European countries, health psychology is often used as a label for secondary and tertiary prevention with regard to patients with organic and/or psychogenic disorders. The area of primary prevention in the health and medical field is only just beginning to be of interest for psychologists. At the moment, first steps towards the development of a curriculum for the training in health psychology or public health are being taken.

Health education and health promotion

The review of health education by Marsen-Storz, Neuhaus and Robertz-Grossmann (1988) concentrates mainly on the structure and activities of

1) the Federal Centre for Health Information ("Bundeszentrale für gesundheitliche Aufklärung", BZgA) and

2) the Central Agency for Health Education ("Bundesvereinigung für Gesundheitserziehung"),the umbrella organisation for non-governmental health education initiatives.

According to their own description, "the services provided by the BZgA should help individual citizens to take more responsibility for their own health and for the health of those around them. They should also be educated to use the health service correctly. The main principle governing all health education activities is that they must help the citizens to help themselves." (p. 105) They identify as their current priorities, AIDS-related education, non-smoking campaigns and training for public health authorities and, as their future priority campaigns, the promotion of women's health and of health-related self-help.

Special models and projects in the health promotion area include some projects which are mainly focusing on the prevention of cardiovascular diseases, e.g., the German cardiovascular prevention study and the "7 against 7" (meaning, 7 actions to prevent 7 diseases) (cf., Bundesvereinigung für Gesundheitserziehung, 1986; Laaser et al., 1987; Schäfer & Wachtel, 1989; Stark, 1989; Wengle, 1984; Wiesemann, 1990).

The regional health insurance system AOK in Mettmann (cf., Bindzius & Rosenbaum, 1989) focuses on the prevention of coronary heart disease with an interdisciplinary approach. Five health centers with interdisciplinary teams have been created. Their behaviour therapy-oriented program includes individual counseling, information, and other activities focusing on weight problems, lack of exercise, smoking, stress, and psychosocial factors.

A few research projects have been initiated by universities. The Special Research Center in Bielefeld granted by the German Research Association is concerned with prevention and intervention in childhood and adolescence.

Based on the WHO's concepts "Health 2000" and "Healthy Cities", several community projects have been started by federal, state or local organizations (e.g., Bundesvereinigung für Gesundheitserziehung, 1986; Hildebrandt & Trojan, 1988; Stark, 1989; Wilm & Jork, 1987).

4.2.2 (Former) GERMAN DEMOCRATIC REPUBLIC

Although the German Democratic Republic does not exists as a separate country any more, the state of health psychology before the "unification" will be described because of its historical and political importance.

Health system

The description and evaluation of the health system and of health education before the November '89 "revolution" in the GDR in comparison with the re-evaluation to date provides a good example of the dependence of the field on political systems and the structure of the health system in general. It also shows the importance of the source of information about such fields which strongly rely on basic attitudes and values.

According to the WHO (1989),

> "the WHO strategy and the health policy aims of the German Democratic Republic are closely matched and complement each other particularly well . . . Primary health care is available to the entire population . . . 20% of the funds allocated to health care in 1987 were assigned to community care . . . Medical care is provided to all women during pregnancy and childbirth to all infants . . . 94% of live-born infants had a birth weight of 2500g or over . . . There is an organized system for reporting information on environmental hazards, and the reports on indicators in the national strategy form part of the national health service reporting system."

The structure of the health system will not to be described in detail (see Institut für Medizinische Statistik und Datenverarbeitung, 1988; WHO, 1989). For a broad overview it should be mentioned that it was a socialist health system with totally free health care and very few physicians in private practice. At the moment the system is being adapted to the structures of the FRG's system (cf., Arnold & Schirmer, 1990), e.g. putting more emphasis on physicians in private practice instead of polyclinics.

Health psychology

According to the report by Ludwig, Schmidt, and Lämmel (1988) the area of health education seemed to be very well developed in the GDR at that time.

At the 7th National Conference on Health Education in 1983 the minister of health indicated the main directions and emphases:

> "1) Active efforts to safeguard peace as the most important factor of protecting life and health . . .
>
> 2) Promotion of healthy behavior in personal life in order to stabilise and encourage adaptability and efficiency . . .
>
> 3) Creation of healthy working and living conditions through the participation of the citizen . . .
>
> 4) Support of the socialist health services , medical, special and preventive measures by persuading

and enabling the citizen to behave understandingly and receptively towards preventive measures, and, in the case of illness, by allowing correct first aid and home nursing care." (Ludwig, Schmidt, & Lämmel, 1988, p. 92)

As example for an "effective method of stimulating scientific studies" several symposia were organized by the Institute for Health Education (cf., Ludwig, Schmidt, & Lämmel, 1988).

Since, in health psychology, the goals, objectives and evaluations are mostly described in an ideological and political manner, they are extremely likely to become integrated parts of political systems with similar foci. This applies especially to socialist countries where the declarations within the areas of health psychology correspond remarkably with the WHO's programmes and evaluations. This becomes obvious in Reschke's (1990) documentation of health related topics in the GDR journal "Humanitas" from 1987 to 1989.

This explains why the current rapid changes of the health system in the GDR will not depend on rational and differentiated analyses of different health systems (cf., Gruppe Demokratie für Gesundheit, 1990; Anonymous, 1990) or health system indicators (cf., Alber, 1988, 1989) but on ideologic, political or economic considerations.

4.4 SPAIN

Health system

Miguel and Guillén (1989) describe the Spanish health system (Sistema Nacional de Salud) as follows:

"The public sector is organized into concentric rings: state administration, health services of regional administrations, health areas, and basic health zones. At each level a health planning mechanism is designed, which is then combined with ones from other levels to form a Plan Integrado de Salud (PIS) or Integrated Health Plan. The population participates merely as a consultative organism and always in a minority position." (Miguel & Guillén, 1989, p. 160).

In their evaluation, they criticize this system as

" . . . (1) unbalanced (too many physicians, too few beds); (2) disorganized, fragmented, and sometimes chaotic; (3) subsidiary to private interests (those of the professions, the pharmaceutical sector, and the multinationals); (4) concentrated in an expensive hospital health care system, compared to primary health care; and (5) lacking adequate planning, but which paradoxically still allows favourable health levels." (p. 160)

The "general lack of hospital beds" and the fact that "only 9.2% of the population is admitted to a hospital each year" are from our point of view not necessarily to be considered as flaws in a health system – the rather high levels of health status (cf., Alber, 1988) seem to indicate the contrary.

As possible explanations for the high health levels in Spain, Miguel and Guillén (1989) mention: (1) a low proportion of women working; (2) high urbanization rates; (3) good basic health education of the population; and (4) the traditional Spanish diet. These "explanations" seem to be quite arbitrary and their value is weakened further by their own statement that, on the other hand, housing and sanitary equipment are deficient and consumption of pork, alcohol and tobacco are high. Furthermore,

"these high health levels are however unevenly distributed. Health inequalities are even more obvious than the high health level. Variables such as social class, sex, age, rural/urban strata, and province of residence underlie a structure in which not all the population shares the same health level; and only a small proportion may participate in health planning." (Miguel and Guillén, 1989, p. 162).

Health psychology

The evaluation of the state of health psychology in general by Fernandez-Ballesteros and Carrobles (1989) is quite optimistic. They mention two post-graduate programmes in health psychology (at the University Autonoma of Madrid and at the University of Valencia). Thirteen Health Promotion Services (CPS) governed by the Madrid City Council were organised with the explicit goals of health promotion and prevention services. The staff of each CPS should include two psychologists. Eight psychologists work in the national health clinics, and a new journal of health psychology ("Revista de Psicologia de la Salud") has been established. Furthermore, an institute has been created to enhance the application of research in regional health planning. This institute is structured to integrate several functions by combining diverse roles in research, the development of health promotion strategies, the coordination of action for health promotion, and the development of appropriate personnel for both general health services and health promotion (cf., Martinez & Peruga, 1988).

Also promising are the descriptions of *health promotion* and *health education* by the WHO (1989) and the IUHE author Najera (1988). Najera (1988) emphasises the development of health education services in the Autonomous Communities, offering professionals opportunities for training and working in this area and possibilities for financing health education programmes. However, the administrative structure for the development of health education is being described as "deficient", both at state and at regional level.

The integration of health education in the general school system has been promoted by the Ministry of Education and Science and the Ministry of Health and Consumer Affairs as well as by several Autonomous Communities.

The main drawback of mass media health education in Spain can be seen in the contribution to the medicalisation of society and the tendency to focus more on disease and prevention than on health and its promotion. Research in health education has been restricted to surveys on attitudes and behaviour in relation to the use of food, tobacco, alcohol and on health knowledge or risk factors. Little is being investigated on health education methodology and the effects of the integration of health education in different programmes.

4.5 SWEDEN

Health system

The Swedish Government promptly provided thorough information about their health system and health education and health promotion efforts. According to their fact sheet on the health system, the fundamental principle of the Swedish welfare system is that all citizens are entitled to good health and have equal access to health and medical care, regardless of where they live and their economic circumstances. Health and medical care is seen as a public sector responsibility which is supported by a national health insurance system. This insurance system is a principal means of creating socioeconomic equality while also functioning as a financing instrument and one of state control and supervision.

Responsibility for health and medical care, both inpatient and outpatient, is a duty of the 23 county councils and three large municipalities. Outpatient care is organized into *primary care districts*. At the health centres, district physicians, normally general practitioners but sometimes also specialists, provide medical treatment, advisory services and preventive care. The outpatient system also includes district nurses and midwives and runs clinics for child and maternity health care. County level medical care covers patients with critical conditions or other illnesses requiring access to staff or technical resources which, for various reasons, must be concentrated in one or a few hospitals within each county council area.

Private health care exists on a limited scale. Only about 5% of the physicians work full-time in private practice. For patients, there is no free choice of physicians since this is the responsibility of the physician in the region where one lives. Physicians are usually paid with a fixed salary. Keil et al. (1990) are quite critical of this system, especially with regard to the primary health care (practitioners) and their poor cooperation with physicians in the hospitals.

Sweden excells with regard to most criteria of a good health system. Although it is extremely expensive, the Swedish health system is extremely socialist with regard to equality of services. In its declaration "The Swedish health services in the 1990's", the National Board of Health and Welfare (1985) emphasizes that health care must be secured on equal terms for the entire population. However, the role of the non-governmental organizations and the participation of citizens seems to grow according to the overview on health promotion by Eklundh and Pettersson (1987).

Health psychology

According to the IUHE review by Lindvall (1988), the Swedish Parliament has laid down four goals for health education:

"— to increase public knowledge of prevailing health risks and create a better understanding of ways of developing healthier living habits;

— to provide guidance for action on an individual level;

— to bring about greater health awareness on the part of the public;

— to establish clearly the links between ill-health and social and environmental conditions." (p. 218)

As in many other countries, these general propositions sound very convincing but need to be realized and reflected in specific actions and financial support. There appear to be promising developments in the fields of health promotion (cf., Eklundh & Pettersson, 1987) and public health (cf., National Board of Health and Welfare, 1985). A significant change towards prevention and health promotion has taken place during the last decade in Swedish health policy. In 1987, trained personnel within the health system included 23.600 physicians and 5.000 psychologists (although probably mainly not working in "true" health psychology). A resolution of Parliament started national health programmes against cardiovascular disease, cancer and accidental injury in 1985. Health education programmes dealing with smoking, dietary habits, sexually transmitted diseases, alcohol, drugs, physical exercise and other health risk areas of concern are being planned. Special aims are to strengthen people's chances of influencing health policies and community planning, to foster health education in the school system, to improve the health education training of health personnel and to increase the efforts in epidemiological research and intervention studies. Several pilot projects are planned or have already started) such as the one in the Västerbotton County Council which focuses on preventing cardiovascular disease and diabetes or the one in Stockholm which focuses on prevention of cancer by smoking cessation and dietary improvement (Lindvall, 1988).

4.6 UNITED KINGDOM

Health system

Johnston (1990) describes the main features of the British health system as follows: "The National Health Service (NHS), established in 1948, provides the full range of health services to all citizens of the UK with no charge at the point of delivery of service. The service is funded via taxation administered by the Department of Health and Social Security which is the responsibility of the Minister of Health, a senior minister in the Government. It is therefore subject to direct political influence both in determining funds available and how these are spent . . . Within the NHS, each individual is encouraged to be registered with a general medical practitioner (GP), who provides primary medical care, is the first point of access to NHS facilities and makes referals to other specialist services." (p. 8ff.)

In his comprehensive overview, Chester (1984) summarizes:

"The National Health Service in Great Britain is viewed abroad as a vast monolithic organisation, employing one and a quarter million staff with a total current expenditure of approximately DM 80 milliards . . . The reality of its operation is very different. It is located within a democratic society with a long history permitting the exercise of participation in decision-making at many points . . . " (p. 199).

UK is spending much less money on the health sector than other comparable European countries. One has to wonder if therefore certain costs are not accounted for, whether special services and equipment resources (e.g., CT-scanners: Alber, 1989) are not provided sufficiently, or whether other countries might be overequipped. The social aspects of the system (free care as well as for example self help groups) seem to be quite well developed but some services (especially in the social field) seem outdated and no longer adequate for the living standard of the population (e.g., Keil et al., 1990). One example for saving costs in the UK is the exclusion of many elderly people from hemodialysis. Alber (1989) sees this to be supported by physicians who translate economic requirements into medical arguments such as the painfulness or stressfulness of the treatment.

Health psychology

According to Johnston (1990), "health psychology in the UK is very buoyant and developing with exciting momentum" (p. 10).

The NHS employs about 2.000 clinical psychologists who are usually employed by a District to provide services to a specified population. These services may be delivered in hospital, clinic or community settings. During the last 15 years, services have moved increasingly to the community, and many clinical psychologists work at least partially in primary care settings (cf., Johnston, 1990).

In England one in 5–7 psychologists is working with general practitioners (Diekstra, 1990). Each GP has a registered list of 2.000 to 2.500 patients and may work in collaboration with a primary care team which can include nurses, counsellors, psychologists, etc. (cf., Johnston, 1990).

"However, the developments have largely occured in the last 10 years and have occured with little additional funding. Current constraints in Government spending, both in the NHS and in Education, may limit developments and prevent health psychology making its full potential." (Johnston, 1990, p. 10)

550 members of the British Psychological Society belong to the Health Psychology Section. According to Johnston (1990), almost all of these are employed in the public sector, about half in Universities or Polytechnics and half by the NHS. Less than 1% of health psychologists work exclusively in the private sector.

Health education

The situation in the field of health education in the UK might best be reflected by Jacob (1988):

"New opportunities for health education are continually arising as the field expands and diversifies. Health education now has workers in industry, local authorities, schools, universities and colleges, adult education, and professional training . . . health education has moved firmly into the mainstream of society, and is now so much part of daily life, that it can easily be forgotten how far things have developed since the Health Education Council was founded in 1968 . . . However, the prospects for health are not all encouraging. Reports have indicated that the health of people in Britain is falling behind that of the rest of Europe, and that the gap between rich and poor, and access to health services, is widening . . . The challenges do not diminish, but experience shows that education, allied with a determination to affect and shape public policy and, if necessary, to engage in economic arguments, can be both effective, and cost-effective." (p. 246ff.)

5. HEALTH PSYCHOLOGY IN EUROPE: DISCUSSION AND OUTLOOK

Evaluating the current state of health psychology in Europe does not leave us with a very encouraging picture. At the moment, health psychology in Europe generally is – at least in practice and education – underdeveloped and therefore a differentiated conclusion is not really possible. This is remarkable because the political and cultural backgrounds of the different European countries and therefore also the health systems are very heterogeneous in structure and organization.

Recently, some developments towards a European health psychology have taken place. Since 1986 the European Health Psychology Society has organized annual conferences of health psychology in varying European countries (cf., Maes, Spielberger, Defares & Sarason, 1988; Schmidt, Schwenkmezger, Weinman, & Maes, 1990). Increasingly, international and national conferences in Europe include health psychology symposia and "Psychology & Health", an international journal in this field, was founded in 1986. Training in health psychology is developing (see Methorst, Jansen & Kerkhof, 1990) and some universities in the Netherlands and in the United Kingdom already offer a master's program in health psychology. The "Erasmus" program (an international exchange program for students from EC countries) has established a health psychology program for post graduate students. Even if not all the developments strictly reflect health psychology in our sense, this label is increasingly being used and the "Zeitgeist" seems to be directed towards health and primary prevention.

In order to discuss the status of health psychology in Europe different kinds of prerequisites have to be carefully considered. In most countries a valid report about the status of health psychology is not available. Data from varying sources have to be gathered from different disciplines. Additionally, it is very hard to decide how objective, reliable and valid the data are. Furthermore, as was discussed above, at the moment there is no agreement about the topics which health psychology should be concerned with. This can lead to misinterpretation of publications, such as that done by Stone (1990) who used mainly Dahme and Scheer's (1986) review about medical psychology in Germany in his report to describe the state of health psychology there.

Important indicators for health psychology have to include psychological and social as well as ecological indicators which are not investigated enough. There is a particular lack of indicators for psychological aspects of health, such as life style, well-being, functions of risk factors or coping strategies.

The focus on economic aspects is too restricted even with regard to indicators of the physical health status and life expectancy. Krämer (1989) claims for example that from a statistical point of view a longer life expectancy is correlated with higher health expenditure (e.g., because of an increasing incidence of diseases such as cancer or heart diseases). This is more the case when considering psychosocial aspects of primary prevention and there is currently considerable debate about the cost-effectiveness of prevention (e.g., Borgers, 1989; DeFriese, 1986; Doerken & DeLeon, 1986; Field, 1989a, b; Krämer, 1989; McCaughrin, 1984; Russell, 1986).

Health psychology has to develop other goals than the mere prevention of disease or even the reduction of costs caused by them as for example Taylor (1990) claims:

"Subtly, the pressures of cost containment push us in the direction of research questions designed to keep people out of the health care system altogether. On the clinical and practice side, interventions increasingly examine the benefits and liabilities of self-help groups, peer counseling, self-management programs such as those for hemodialysis . . . , and other inexpensive ways to provide service delivery to those who might otherwise not receive care." (pp. 46)

Health psychology also needs to focus on other issues such as quality of life, well-being or reinforcing aspects of prevention. One main problem of prevention seems to be that its positive consequences are often indirect and only seen in the long run. This might partially explain the lack of political, legal or financial support. Some authors emphasize that besides individual changes towards health promotion a "new environmental ethic" respectively a "health care revolution" is needed (cf., Michael, 1983; Kiesler & Morton, 1988).

"A new epidemiology of everyday health actions might suggest new priorities for allocating resources for preventive care and supportive services. In the framework of this new epidemiology, 'healthy life-style' would no longer focus on individual 'risk factor reduction' but on new definitions of significant health actions and health potential." (Kickbusch, 1988, p. 242)

In this context various ethical aspects of primary prevention in the health field have to be considered. One important question is the setting of norms for a health promoting life style – for the individual (subjective well-being, psychological and social functions of risk behaviours) as well as for whole cultural backgrounds (especially with regard to the heterogeneity of the different European countries). Other crucial aspects are concerned with the decision about the responsibility to maintain health and the scientific data on which suggestions for life-style changes are based. It is important however, not to "blame the victims" for their diseases:" . . . a person may not be responsible for being sick, but he or she is responsible for doing something about it" (Ullman, 1988, p. 72).

In conclusion, the concept of healthy life style must be examined more closely. We need a new concept of 'normality', social policies which reward healthy behaviour instead of compensating for illness a posteriori, methods for treating the community as a system for formal and informal relations as such, and to "assess urgently how the so-called health system does in fact work to produce full health by avoiding negative, unattended, or perverse outcomes." (Donati, 1988, p. 250)

The question of *supply and demand* of services in health psychology still needs to be solved (see also Gäfgen, 1988; Paffrath, 1986). Therefore, we need to know more about what to offer and how to offer it. The focus should become primary prevention in physical *and* mental health. However, individuals should be free to decide how to use health promotion services. It is important that they are neither forced into health behaviour nor sanctioned for risk behaviours (e.g., by law). This does not necessarily hold true for extreme cases who are endangering their own or other lives (see for example the controversial discussions regarding AIDS or infection with HIV).

Health psychology services should in principle be available for everybody and for healthy subpopulations (for example at the worksite) and for populations with certain risk behaviors or in certain risk groups, respectively. Whenever possible, these services should be provided in cooperation with other professions, institutions and organisations. The special contributions of psychologists in these teams might be manifold. In general, they should use psychological methods and knowledge on the basis of models of health, health behavior or health promotion, thus including the functional and practical implications of these approaches (cf., Dlugosch & Schmidt, in preparation). Particularly, they could rely on psychological functions and processes (such as communication, motivation, social group processes, risk behavior, coping, critical ecological conditions or critical phases in life span development, etc.) as well as on strategies and methods of assessment and intervention. A crucial question is when, where and how changes can be induced and maintained and who sets the norms for these interventions. Health psychologists may accept the promotion of health and well-being as general targets but they should neither become the compliance specialists for (health) goals of other professions or society nor should they keep people away from the benefits of medicine (cf., Taylor, 1990). On the other hand, as Borgers (1989) discusses, prevention has also to prevent people from potential damage by medicine.

In most European countries the demand for health psychology is not great and there is not usually the insurance coverage or legal basis for psychological services. Psychologists are still mainly seen as experts for psychopathology. This is one more reason to develop separate concepts and services for clinical psychology and for health psychology.

This leads us to some reflections about the professional issues in the health field. First to be mentioned is the power struggle between the medical and other professions in the health system that impedes developments of disciplines like psychology and especially health psychology. For example, physicians claim to also be responsible for health promotion even though their job is to diagnose and treat diseases and they are usually not trained in counseling or psychological interventions.

On the other hand, psychologists need to demonstrate how they can be valuable in the above mentioned goals (reducing costs; decreasing hospital admissions and physician consultations; improving health status and well-being). First steps in this direction have been taken especially in the USA as documented by Bühringer and Hahlweg (1986) or Rosen and Wiens (1979). Further objectives on a theoretical basis should involve the development of health models and health promotion models together with the design and evaluation of intervention studies and pilot projects.

We do not want to finish this chapter without having acknowledged that our strict definition of health psychology leads to the exclusion of very many valuable results of medical and clinical psychology in research and practice. Nevertheless, this strong position seems necessary in order to induce important changes within the given health systems (e.g., increasing the proportion of expenditure for preventive services). Even more important but also more challenging would appear to be the creation of a real health system that does not only focus on illness, treatment, secondary and tertiary prevention but also understands the promotion and maintenance of health as a task for the whole society. As a relatively young discipline, health psychology has not yet been able to develop the scientific basis and the power to induce such changes. Hopefully, the current dramatic political and structural changes in Europe will also lead to improvements of the health systems and that health psychologists will take a leading position within this process.

References

Alber, J. (1988). Die Gesundheitssysteme der OECD-Länder im Vergleich [Comparison of the health systems of the OECD countries]. In M. G. Schmidt (Ed.), *Staatstätigkeit. Politische Vierteljahresschrift Sonderheft* **19.** Opladen: Westdeutscher Verlag.

Alber, J. (1989). Die Steuerung des Gesundheitswesens in vergleichender Perspektive [Steering of health systems in comparison]. *Journal für Sozialforschung*, **29,** 259–284.

Anonymous. (1990). *Das Gesundheits- und Sozialwesen in der DDR* [The health and social system in the GDR]. Krankenhaus Umschau 2/90, p. 95.

Arnold, M., and Schirmer, B. (1990). *Gesundheit für ein Deutschland.* [Health for one Germany]. Köln: Deutscher Ärzte Verlag.

Bindzius, F. and Rosenbaum, M. (1989). 10 Jahre Aktion Gesundheit – Zwischenbilanz und Reflexion eines interdisziplinären Präventionskonzeptes [10 years action health – interim report and reflection about an interdisciplinary concept of prevention]. *Report Psychologie*, **43,** 16–25.

Borgers, D. (1989). *Epidemiologie und Gesundheitswissenschaft*, [Epidemiology and the science of health]. Berlin: Argument.

Buchholz, E. H. (Ed.). (1988). *Das Gesundheitswesen in der Bundesrepublik Deutschland* [The health care system of the Federal Republic of Germany]. Berlin: Springer.

Bühringer, G. and Hahlweg, L. (1986). Kosten-Nutzen Aspekte psychologischer Behandlung [Cost-benefit aspects of psychological treatment]. *Psychologische Rundschau*, **37,** 1–19.

Bundesgesundheitsamt. (Ed.). (1989). *Tätigkeitsbericht 1988*, [Report 1988]. München: MMV Medizin Verlag.

Bundesminister für Jugend, Familie, Frauen und Gesundheit. (1988). *Das Gesundheitswesen in der Bundesrepublik Deutschland*, [The health system in the FRG]. Kiel: Schmidt and Klaunig.

Bundesvereinigung für Gesundheitserziehung (Ed.). (1986). *Gemeindenahe Gesundheitserziehung*,[Community based health education]. Regensburg: Mittelbayerische Druckerei.

Chester, T. E. (1984). A public health system in a democratic society: A case study of the British National Health Service. In G. Neubauer (Ed.), *Alternativen der Steuerung des Gesundheitswesens im Rahmen einer sozialen Marktwirtschaft*, (pp. 199–231). Gerlingen : Bleicher.

Dahme, B. and Scheer, J. (1986). Medical psychology in the Federal Republic of Germany. *Advances*, **3,** 19–35.

DeFriese, G. H. (1986). Cost effectiveness as a basis for assessing the policy significance of health promotion. *Advances in Health Education and Promotion*, **1,** 7–21.

Deppe, H.-U. (Ed.). (1983). *Gesundheitssysteme und Gesundheitspolitik in Westeuropa*, [Health care systems and health policy in Western Europe]. Frankfurt: Campus.

Deppe, H.-U. and Lenhardt, U. (1990). *Westeuropäische Integration und Gesundheitspolitik*, [Western European integration and health politics]. Marburg: Verlag Arbeit und Gesellschaft.

Diekstra, R. F. W. (1990). Psychology, health and health care. *Psychology and Health,* **4,** 51–63.

Diekstra, R. F. W. and Jansen, M. A. (1990). The importance of psychological intervention in primary health care. In L. R. Schmidt, P. Schwenkmezger, J. Weinman, and S. Maes (Eds.), *Theoretical and applied aspects of health psychology*, (pp. 87–102). Chur: Harwood.

Dlugosch, G. E. and Schmidt, L. R. (in preparation). Gesundheitspsychologie [Health psychology]. In R. Bastine (Ed.) *Klinische Psychologie. Band 2.*

Doerken, H. and DeLeon, P. H. (1986). Cost as the driving force in health care reform. In H. Doerken and Associates (Eds.). *Professional psychology in transition*, (pp. 313–349). San Francisco: Jossey-Bass.
Donati, P. (1988). The need for new social perspectives in health-behaviour research. In R. Anderson, J. K. Davies, I. Kickbusch, D. v. McQueen, and J. Turner (Eds.), *Health behaviour research and health promotion*, (pp. 244–250). Oxford. Oxford University Press.
Eklundh, B. and Pettersson, B. (1987). Health promotion policy in Sweden: Means and methods in intersectoral action. *Health Promotion*, **2,** 177–194.
Fernandez-Ballesteros, R. and Carrobles, J. A. I. (1989). Spain. In M. Johnston (Ed.), *Health psychology in Europe*. Unpublished manuscript.
Field, M. G. (Ed.). (1989a). *Success and crisis in national health systems: A comparative approach*. New York: Routledge.
Field, M. G. (1989b). Comparative evolution of health systems: Convergence, diversity and cross-cutting issues. In G. Lüschen, W. C. Cockerham, and G. Kunz (Eds.), *Health and illness in America and Germany*, (pp. 15–30). München: Oldenbourg.
Forgács, I. and Kökény, M. (1989). *Health, health care, social services*. Budapest: Turbo GM.
Gäfgen, G (Ed.). (1986). *Ökonomie des Gesundheitswesens*, [Economy of the health care system]. Berlin: Duncker and Humblot.
Gäfgen, G. (1988). Gesundheitspolitik als Verteilungspolitik, [Health politics as distribution politics]. *MMG*, **13,** 95–108.
Gäfgen, G. and Lampert, H. (Eds.). (1982). *Beiträge zur Gesundheitsökonomie. Band 3: Betrieb, Markt und Kontrolle im Gesundheitswesen*, [Issues of health economy, Vol. 3: Management, market, and control within the health care system]. Gerlingen: Bleicher.
Gruppe Demokratie für Gesundheit. (1990). *Gesundheitssystemgestaltung*, [Designing health care systems]. Unpublished manuscript.
Harris, P. R. (1980). *Promoting health-preventing disease: Objectives for the nation*. Washington, D.C.: US Government Printing Office.
Hildebrandt, H. and Trojan, A. (1988). *Gesündere Zukunft für Hamburg*, [A healthier future for Hamburg]. Hamburg: Sozialwissenschaften und Gesundheit.
Institut für Medizinische Statistik und Datenverarbeitung. (Ed.). (1988). *Das Gesundheitswesen DDR 1988*, [The health system GDR 1988]. Berlin: Hectography.
International Union for Health Education. (Ed.). (1988). *Health education in Europe – State of the art of health education in 28 European countries*. Utrecht: The Dutch Health Education Centre.
Jacob, M. (1988);. United Kingdom/England. In International Union for Health Education (Ed.), *Health education in Europe – State of the art of health education in 28 European countries*, (pp. 245–252). Utrecht: The Dutch Health Education Centre.
Johnston, M. (1990). Health psychology in Europe: United Kingdom. *EHPS Newsletter,* **1,** 7–10.
Juusela, T. (1988). Finland. In International Union for Health Education (Ed.), *Health education in Europe – State of the art of health education in 28 European countries*, (pp. 63–75). Utrecht: The Dutch Health Education Centre.
Kalimo, E. (1988). National surveys of health behaviour in Finland. In R. Anderson, J. K. Davies, I. Kickbusch, D. v. McQueen, and J. Turner (Eds.), *Health behaviour research and health promotion*, (pp. 125–136). Oxford: Oxford University Press.
Keil, W., Migenda, A., Mittag, D., Münch, A., Nitzschke, M., Zimmer, F. and Friedemann, H. (1990). *Systemvergleich zum Gesundheits- und Sozialwesen ausgewählter Länder*, [Comparison of health and social systems in selected countries]. Berlin: Hectography.
Kickbusch, I. (1988). New perspectives for research in health behaviour. In R. Anderson, J. K. Davies, I. Kickbusch, D. v. McQueen, and J. Turner (Eds.), *Health behaviour research and health promotion*, (pp. 237–243). Oxford University Press.
Kiesler, C. A. and Morton, T. L. (1988). Psychology and public policy in the "health care revolution". *American Psychologist*, **43,** 993–1003.
Koch, E. R., Klopfleisch, R. and Maywald, A. (1986). *Die Gesundheit der Nation*, [The health of the nation]. Köln: Kiepenheuer & Witsch.
Krämer, W. (1989). *Die Krankheit des Gesundheitswesens. Die Fortschrittsfalle der modernen Medizin*, [The illness of the health care system – the progress pitfalls of modern medicine]. Frankfurt: Fischer.
Laaser, U., Sassen, G., Murza, G. and Sabo, P. (Eds.). (1987). *Prävention und Gesundheitserziehung*, [Prevention and health education]. Berlin: Springer.
Lindvall, I. (1988). Sweden. In International Union for Health Education (Ed.), *Health education in Europe – State of the art of health education in 28 European countries*, (pp. 217–224). Utrecht: The Dutch Health Education Centre.
Ludwig, W., Schmidt, W. and Lämmel, R. (1988). German Democratic Republic. In International Union

for Health Education (Ed.), *Health education in Europe – State of the art of health education in 28 European countries*, (pp. 89–102). Utrecht: The Dutch Health Education Centre.
Maes, S., Spielberger, C. D., Defares, P. B. and Sarason, I. G. (Eds.). (1988). *Topics in health psychology*. Chichester: Wiley.
Marsen-Storz, G., Neuhaus, G. and Robertz-Grossmann, B. (1988). German Federal Republic. In International Union for Health Education (Ed.), *Health education in Europe – State of the art of health education in 28 European countries*, (pp. 103–119). Utrecht: The Dutch Health Education Centre.
Martinez, R. and Peruga, A. (1988). The autonomous region of Madrid. In R. Anderson, J. K. Davies, I. Kickbusch, D. v. McQueen, and J. Turner (Eds.), *Health behaviour research and health promotion*, (pp. 200–206). Oxford: Oxford University Press.
Matarazzo, J. D. (1980). Behavioural health and behavioral medicine – Frontiers for a new health psychology. *American Psychologist*, **35,** 807–817.
Matarazzo, J. D., Weiss, J. M., Herd, J. A., Miller, N. E. and Weiss, S. M. (Eds.). (1984). *Behavioral health – A handbook of health enhancement and disease prevention*, New York: Wiley.
Maynard, A. (1982). *Health care in the European Community*, London: Croom Helm.
McCaughrin, W. C. (1984). Dollars and sense: The economics of personal health decision-making. *Health Policy*, **4,** 101–116.
Methorst, G. J., Jansen, M. A. and Kerkhof, A. J. F. M. (1990). Training in health psychology: An international look. *Psychology and Health*, **4,** 19–30.
Michael, J. M. (1982). The second revolution in health. *American Psychologist*, **37,** 936–941.
Miguel, J. M. and Guillén, M. F. (1989). The health system in Spain. In M. G. Field (Ed.), *Success and crisis in national health systems: A comparative approach*, (pp. 128–164). New York: Routledge.
Najera, P. (1988). Spain. In International Union for Health Education (Ed.), *Health education in Europe – State of the art of health education in 28 European countries*, (pp. 207–216). Utrecht: The Dutch Health Education Centre.
National Board of Health and Welfare. (1985). *The Swedish Health Services in the 1990s*. Stockholm: The National Board of Health and Welfare.
OECD (1990). *Health care systems in transition*, Paris:. OECD.
Paffrath, D. (1986). Ist eine angebotsorientierte Nachfrage im Gesundheitswesen notwendig? [Is a supply-oriented demand necessary in the health system?] In H. Silomon, R. Breunecke, C. von Ferber, and U. Laaser (Eds.), *Sozialmedizin, Sozialrecht, Gesundheitsökonomie*, (pp. 87–99). Berlin: Springer.
Puska, P. (1984). Community-based prevention of cardiovascular disease: The North Karelia project. In J. D. Matarazzo, J. M. Weiss, J. A. Herd, N. E. Miller, and S. M. Weiss (Eds.), *Behavioral health – A handbook of health enhancement and disease prevention*, (pp. 1140–1147). New York: Wiley.
Reschke, K. (1990). Leitsymptom Gesundheit [Leading symptom health]. Unpublished manuscript.
Rimpelä, M., Rimpelä, A., Rahkonen, O. and Teperi, J. (1988). The evolution of the juvenile health habit study 1977–1985. In R. Anderson, J. K. Davies, I. Kickbusch, D. v. McQueen, and J. Turner (Eds.), *Health behaviour research and health promotion*, (pp. 154–171). Oxford: Oxford University Press.
Rosen, J. C. and Wiens, A. N. (1979). Changes in medical problems and use of medical services following psychological intervention. *American Psychologist*, **34,** 420–431.
Russell, L. B. (1986). *Is prevention better than cure?* Washington: The Brookings Institution.
Schach, E. (Ed.). (1985). *Von Gesundheitsstatistiken zu Gesundheitsinformation*, [From health statistics to health information]. Berlin: Springer.
Schäfer, T. and Wachtel, H.-W. (1989). *Umweltbezogene Gesundheitsberichterstattung – Planungsstudie*, [Environmental health reporting – a planning study]. Sankt Augustin: Asgard Verlag.
Schmidt, L. R., Schwenkmezger, P., Weinman, J. and Maes, S. (1990). *Theoretical and applied aspects of health psychology*, Chur: Harwood.
Schmidt, L. R., Schwenkmezger, P. and Dlugosch, G. E. (1990). The scope of health psychology. In L. R. Schmidt, P. Schwenkmezger, J. Weinman and S. Maes (Eds.), *Theoretical and applied aspects of health psychology*, (pp. 3–28). Chur: Harwood.
Schmidt, U. (1983). *Kosteneinflußfaktoren im Gesundheitswesen* [Factors influencing costs in the health care system]. Frankfurt: Lang.
Schneider, M. (1990). Strukturdaten der Gesundheitssysteme in der EG. [Structural data of the health systems in the EG]. *MMG*, **15,** 66–75.
Schwefel, D. (Ed.). (1987). *Indicators and trends in health and health care*. Berlin: Springer.
Stark, W. (1989). *Lebensweltbezogene Prävention und Gesundheitsförderung – Konzepte und Strategien für die psychosoziale Praxis.* [Living space centered prevention and health promotion – concepts and strategies for the psychosocial practice]. Freiburg: Lambertus.
Stone, G. C. (1990). An international review of the emergence and the development of health psychology.

Psychology and Health, **4,** 3–17.

Taylor, S. E. (1990). Health psychology. The science and the field. *American Psychologist*, **45,** 40–50.

Tietze, U. (1989). *Die gesetzliche Krankenversicherung in der Perspektive von Organisationsreform und EG-Binnenmarkt 1992*, [Health insurance from the perspective of organization changes and the EC-market in 1992]. Hamburg: Unpublished manuscript.

Ullman, D. (1988). Getting beyond wellness macho: The promise and pitfalls of holistic health. *Utne Reader*, (Jan./Feb.), 68–72.

Wengle, E. (Ed.). (1984). *Modellversuch Gesundheitsberatungsstellen bei der AOK für den Kreis Mettmann*, [The AOK's pilot project for health education centers in the area of Mettmann]. München: Institut für Therapieforschung.

Wiesemann, A. (1990). *Ganzheitliche Wege zur Gesundheit. Neue Chancen für das Arzt-Patienten-Bündnis*, [Holistic ways towards health. New chances for the physician-patient-alliance]. Emsdetten: Chronomed.

Wilm, S. and Jork, K. (1987). Gemeindenahe Prävention – Modelle und Interventionsstrategien am Beispiel einer südhessischen Kleinstadt, [Community based prevention – a southern Hessen town as example for models and intervention strategies]. In K. Jork [Ed.), *Gesundheitsberatung – Einführung und Leitfaden für Ärzte und Studierende der Medizin*, (pp. 191–213). Berlin: Springer.

Winett, R. A., King, A. C. and Altman, D. G. (1989). *Health psychology and public health. An integrative approach*. New York: Pergamon.

World Health Organization. (Ed.). (1987). *Evaluation of the strategy for health for all by the year 2000. Seventh report on the world health situation*. Geneva: WHO.

World Health Organization. (Ed.). (1989). *Monitoring of the strategy for health for all by the year 2000. Part 2: Monitoring by country 1988/1989*. Copenhagen: WHO.

CHAPTER 4

HEALTH PSYCHOLOGY IN AUSTRALIA

BRIAN OLDENBURG

Department of Public Health, University of Sydney, Australia

NEVILLE OWEN†

Department of Community Medicine, University of Adelaide, Australia

Opportunities are expanding rapidly for health psychologists to work in Australia in a wider range of health-care settings, and on challenging aspects of community disease prevention and public health. Published material in psychological journals in Australia does not suggest that there is a trend towards more health psychology research being reported in this country; however, research reported at conferences, and the recent development of specialized research centres, indicate that health psychology is an active and expanding area. Some examples of health psychology research in Australia are presented, and aspects of education and training relevant to health psychology are described.

INTRODUCTION

In this paper we outline recent developments relevant to research and practice in health psychology in Australia. It is not an easy task to give a coherent account of these developments, when there is no single organisation or professional body, such as an equivalent of the Society of Behavioral Medicine or the Psychosomatic Society in the United States, representing the interests of health psychologists and those other health professionals who are involved in these activities.

Australia has a total land area roughly equivalent to that of continental USA, and a population of just over 16 million. Approximately 80% of Australia's population resides in the coastal capital cities of the seven Australian states. Sydney and Melbourne are the most populous cities, with around four million people each; there are six other major urban areas with smaller populations. It is often necessary to travel at least 500 kilometres to the nearest major city. It is almost 5000 kilometres from Perth on the West coast to Sydney on the East coast. Australia has a relatively small population, and most of the population is concentrated in a few urban centres which are distant from one another. Travel for professional and scientific purposes is therefore a relatively time-consuming and expensive undertaking.

Australia has a system of national health insurance, although there has been a recent trend towards "privatisation" of the health care system; it is a system which not only has some of the features of a fully nationalised system such as those found in Scandinavian countries, but also some of the features of highly privatised system such as that found in the USA (Sax, 1984).

† Address correspondence to: Neville Owen, Department of Community Medicine, University of Adelaide, Box 498, Adelaide, Australia 5001.

The Australian Psychological Society (APS), which was a branch of the British Psychological Society until 1966, has a membership of some 5200. The number of Australian psychologists eligible for membership of the APS is estimated to be about 10,000. The APS is the major body representing the professional interests of psychologists in Australia. The APS has boards of clinical neuropsychologists, clinical psychologists, community psychologists, counselling psychologists, educational and developmental psychologists, forensic psychologists and organizational psychologists. Presently, there is no specific health psychology board of the APS; however, in late 1988, the Society established a Working Party on Health Psychology, which will recommend ways to develop the field in Australia. The other society to which many psychologists belong is the Australian Behaviour Modification Association, which was established in the late 1970s. It has a membership of around 800, the majority of whom are psychologists.

Accurate information on the breakdown of numbers of psychologists working in the fields of teaching, research and clinical psychology is not readily available for Australia. There are about 18 Universities which have departments of psychology. But there are a number of universities which are amalgamating, so it is not possible to give exact figures on this.

It is estimated that 70–90% of psychologists employed in Australia are in the public sector. Federal and state governments employ psychologists in education, mental health, community welfare, hospitals and numerous other agencies and services. Academic institutions employ 10 to 20% of psychologists. Of those psychologists providing clinical services in the public sector, most are employed in community mental health or traditional psychiatric settings. With the trend towards de-institutionalisation of psychiatric services, there has been a significant shift in Australia towards transferring inpatient psychiatric facilities away from the traditionally large psychiatric hospitals to smaller inpatient units in general hospitals.

Prior to these changes there were few psychologists engaged in clinical activities within general hospital settings, other than in some of the larger university teaching hospitals. A recent survey of the current activities of psychologists in acute general hospitals in Australia showed that although there were a large number of roles for psychologists in this setting, they were most often restricted to five major treatment areas—neurology, psychosomatic medicine, death and dying, paediatrics and substance abuse (Groth-Marnat, 1988). It is likely that these roles will continue to expand in the future.

In the following section, we describe some recent trends in the development of community-based and preventive health services in Australia, and some ways in which health psychologists have begun to contribute in this area.

Recent Australian Developments in Public Health

Many of the relationships between how people conduct their lives, the interaction of this conduct with social environmental influences, and how this conduct affects their health, are now sufficiently well-established so that epidemiologists and other biomedical scientists are now recommending large-scale, coordinated preventive action (Hetzel and McMichael, 1987). Chronic diseases such as cancer, cardiovascular disease, and adult-onset diabetes have been linked to aspects of "lifestyle," including: cigarette smoking, physical activity patterns, poor dietary practices and stress. We know these risk behaviours are probably important determinants of health and illness (King and Remenyi, 1986). The important issue for psychologists, as it is indeed for other health care professionals, is how to determine to meet the clinical and research needs of the profession so that it is able to participate fully in these new challenges facing the health-care system (Best and Proctor, 1988; Owen and Halford, 1988; Owen and Lee, 1986).

In 1986, the Australian Government established a special commission of health experts and selected laypersons (the Better Health Commission) in order to set Australia's health priorities and to enable health goals from now until the end of the century to be established. The Commission's overall findings (Better Health Commission, 1986) emphasised the importance of community-based, preventive health services; participation by the public in decision-making about health-service priorities; and the explicit consideration of problems of social equity and of access to health services and resources to improve health. These concerns reflect fairly closely those which have come out of reviews and enquiries into the public-health needs of other developed countries (e.g., Califano, 1979).

As a result of the Better Health Commission's work, national, state and local government departments and other funding bodies in Australia have all become significantly more involved in large-scale health promotion initiatives, in which health psychology research has the potential to make significant and extensive contributions. For example, the National Heart Foundation of Australia has recently begun to put more resources into extending the professional and scientific aspects of its own educational and preventive activities; it has also begun to provide more funds to support research and development initiatives in the education and prevention area (e.g., Owen and Dwyer, 1988); to date, psychologists have been reasonably successful in attracting funds from this source. Similarly, State organisations concerned with cancer prevention have been increasing their activities in education and prevention. For example, the Anti-Cancer Council of Victoria has established a Centre for Behavioural Research in Cancer Prevention, staffed by three Ph.D.-level psychologists. It also has a number of research officers with psychology training. The Centre is active in studies of the behavioural epidemiology of cigarette smoking, and trials of methods for smoking cessation with adults and smoking prevention with adolescents; research into compliance issues in screening for breast and cervical cancer is also being carried out.

Recent Developments in Health Psychology in Australia

In a recent survey of individuals involved in health-behaviour research in the Western Pacific region, psychology was found to be the discipline with the greatest representation (32%), followed by medicine (23%), and sociology (14%). The majority of respondents were located in Universities and other centres of tertiary education (70%). The majority of the Australians indicated they had post-graduate qualifications with 47% stating they had acquired a Ph.D. As the context, or target for research, the community was the favoured setting for study (26%), followed by hospital outpatients (15%) and hospital inpatients settings (14%) (Sanson-Fisher, 1984). See Table 1.

The first major Australian conference in the health and behaviour field took place in August, 1980 convened by the Monash University, Department of Psychological Medicine (Tiller and Martin, 1980). Later on that year, Cumberland College of Health Sciences in Sydney hosted the first of a number of behavioural medicine

Table 1 Relative proportions of research activities reported in the health and behaviour area (Sanson-Fisher, 1984)

	Numbers	%
Factors affecting utilization of health services	18	1.2
Aspects of the health care worker patient interaction	115	7.4
Evaluation of health delivery systems	175	11.3
Psychiatric disorder	185	11.9
Health-related legislation	22	1.4
Impact of technological change	3	0.2
Professional issues	243	15.7
Ethical issues	11	0.7
Health economics	26	1.7
Health psychology/health promotion/behavioural factors	754	48.6
TOTAL	1552	100.0

conferences (Sheppard, 1982–87). There are also more generalist conferences at which health psychologists present their work: Australian Psychological Society, the Australian Behaviour Modification Association, the Public Health Association of Australia and New Zealand, the Australian and New Zealand College of Psychiatrists, the Australian Society of Psychiatric Research, and assorted specialist medical conferences.

The type of papers presented at recent Australian conferences and published in local journals is indicative of the activities in this country. An analysis of papers published in the proceedings of the Cumberland College of Health Sciences' Behavioural Medicine conferences for three years (1981–1983) revealed that 14% of papers were on topics related to chronic pain, 13% to issues of occupational health, 13% to chronic/terminal illness and 12% to CHD and risk factors *(Table 2)*.

Dadds (1988) examined the content of papers presented at the last ten national conferences of the Australian Behaviour Modification Association, and of the articles published in the Association's journal, *Behaviour Change,* since its inception in 1984. Health psychology content ranged from less than 20% of all conference papers in 1978 to almost 55% in 1983; however, in 1985, 1986 and 1987, less than one-third of papers have been on health psychology topics. Collapsed across the ten years, less than one quarter of all conference papers were in areas of health psychology, broadly defined. Papers published in the Association's journal, *Beha-*

Table 2 Breakdown of content areas in the proceedings of recent Australian Behavioural Medicine conferences (Sheppard, 1982–87)

Subject area	*Number*	%
Compliance/relapse prevention	5	7
CHD and risk factors	9	12
Chronic pain, headache	11	14
Occupational health	10	13
Obstetrics/gynaecology	5	7
Health care system	6	8
Chronic/terminal illness	10	13
Community-based interventions and health promotion	5	7
Other (doctor–patient communication Aboriginal health, etc.)	15	20

viour Change, showed a similar trend over the years since that journal was first published.

An analysis of the content of articles published in the *Australian Psychologist* (a journal concerned with broad professional, scientific and theoretical issues, published by the Australian Psychological Society) between 1975 and July, 1988 identified some 35 articles which could be described as being in the broad area of health psychology. This was approximately 10% of the total number of articles published in the journal. There was no indication a trend for more health psychology articles in recent years: in 1985 only one such article was published.

These trends in publications in Australian psychology journals, and presentations to conferences, should not be interpreted as suggesting that health psychology is a static area in Australia. A great deal of work on health psychology by Australians is being published in medical journals, or in local and international interdisciplinary medical, public-health, or health psychology journals.

Examples of Australian Health Psychology Research

During the 1960s and 1970s there were many Australian psychologists working in psychiatric and other specialist medical settings. Often, their work was concerned with the evaluation and improvement of medically-oriented approaches to particular diseases in traditional clinical settings. There was a strong tendency until recent years for psychologists in the health field to be affiliated with departments of psychiatry. A number of health psychologists began their research careers working in departments of psychiatry (e.g., Oldenburg, Perkins and Andrews, 1985). Psychologists also formed strong affiliations with other medical specialities, for example, urology (e.g., Millard and Oldenburg, 1983). Collaboration with cardiologists has been a productive area for psychologists (e.g., Oldenburg and Byrne, 1986).

Within the discipline of psychology itself, there have, until recently, been only a small number of departments which have strongly encouraged health psychology research. For example, Lovibond at the University of New South Wales in Sydney has strongly supported a number of health psychology projects (e.g., Lovibond, Birrell and Langeluddecke, 1986); Yates' writings on behaviour therapy were influential while he was at the University of Western Australian (Yates, 1979). Much of the community and preventive work in health psychology has developed out of the concerns for social activism which was implicit in early work on behaviour modification in Australia (Winkler, 1976; Winkler and Krasner, 1987).

Recent work pioneering the application of innovative psychological approaches to many different health problems (see Winkler, 1974) has done a great deal to raise the awareness of medical practitioners about alternatives to psychotropic medication, and to strengthen the consumer-oriented perspective on the actions of health-care providers. Studies have also been conducted on the use of behavioural self-management procedures for sleep problems and asthma, and the application of psychological knowledge to a range of other health problems (Wilson, 1987). Recent research on headache is another example of innovative behavioural-clinical analysis of a major health problem (e.g., Martin, 1986).

King and Remenyi's (1986) book, *Health care: A behavioural approach* gives an overview of much of the health psychology research being done in Australia. The strong influence which North American psychology has had on work in Australia is apparent in this volume. While British and European influences are sometimes apparent, the overwhelming influence seems to be that of the theories and empirical research emanating from behaviour modification and behavioural medicine in the USA.

The future development of health psychology research in Australia will be shaped significantly by the emergence of a critical mass of workers within individual research centres, and in a number of research centres which, ultimately, can collaborate on multi-centre trials and large-scale studies which might require the pooling of data sets.

The Centre for Behavioural Research in Cancer at the Anti-Cancer Council in Victoria, mentioned in an earlier section, has begun to achieve this "critical mass." This Centre has carried out studies of the behavioural epidemiology of smoking, based on data collected nationally (Hill, 1988). A study on the effects of workplace smoking bans, involving researchers in Sydney and Adelaide, is testing a number of hypotheses about the effects of environmental and social determinants of smoking behaviour (Borland, Owen, Chapman and Hill, in press). Work by psychologists at Sydney and Adelaide Universities on a large-scale trial of behavioural intervention techniques to reduce cardiovascular risk in the workplace, funded by the Commonwealth Department of Health, is another example of the collaborative work which is now being developed between a number of Australian health psychologists.

In addition, a number of major research lines in health psychology and behavioural medicine have been developed at the University of Newcastle (e.g. Feletti, Firman and Sanson-Fisher, 1986). These include studies of doctor–patient interaction, diabetes care, screening for various types of cancer, and substance abuse. And, as in many other countries, health psychologists have begun studying the dynamics involved in the transmission of the human immunodeficiency virus (e.g., Ross, 1987).

These examples are far from inclusive of the full range of health psychology research in Australia. There are now a number of centres and departments where psychologists are researching significant health problems in a systematic fashion. Multicentre studies are under way and others are being established, and psychologists are working their way into key positions on national and state health decision-making bodies.

Education and Training in Health Psychology

One of the first health psychology courses was conducted as part of a fourth-year applied diploma programme at the University of Adelaide in the late 1970s. It was taught jointly by a member of the Department of Psychology and a psychologist working in the Medical School (Innes and Owen, 1980). But few Australian university departments of psychology have established curricula for training research and clinical students in health psychology. Although the situation is likely to change in the near future, there is currently no tertiary institution in Australia offering a degree specifically in health psychology at any undergraduate or graduate level (Martin, 1988).

A recent survey (Martin, 1988) showed that, of the 18 University Departments of Psychology in Australia, most had at least some academic staff with an interest in health psychology. Most departments included at least some health psychology material in teaching, offered placements in appropriate settings, and provided opportunities for research in the area. At an undergraduate level, few departments offered extensive or integrated courses in health psychology or related areas.

The courses that now exist are usually half-year courses in the third or fourth years of undergraduate programmes; they are variously labelled "Behavioural Health Management," "Health Psychology," "Behavioural Medicine," or "Behavioural Health Care." Martin (1988) found that the teaching of health psychology is more extensive at graduate level in Australia. The University of Western Australia, University of Adelaide, Curtin University of Technology, La Trobe University, the University of New South Wales, and the University of Sydney all offer units in behavioural medicine or health psychology in their graduate diploma or masters programmes. In the main though, these units are being taught within clinical training programs that are "generalist" rather than "specialist" in their focus.

The Lincoln School of Health Sciences at La Trobe University established a Health Psychology Centre in 1986 which has become very active in teaching, research and consulting activities. The Departments of Psychology and Psychological Medicine, and the Psychology Section of the Faculty of Education at Monash University, have recently established a Centre for Professional Psychology which will offer doctoral training in specialised areas, one of which will be health psychology.

Most undergraduate medical degrees in this country contain some instruction in behavioural medicine or health psychology as part of the behavioural science courses provided during medical students' preclinical years (Sanson-Fisher, 1985; Winefield and Peay, 1980). This teaching is generally carried out by psychologists (and occasionally, by psychiatrists) employed in departments of Psychiatry.

A significant stimulus for research and teaching in those areas of health psychology related to disease prevention and health promotion is coming from Departments of Community Medicine and Public Health in Australian universities. Until 1986 only two universities offered formal graduate courses in public health. By 1988 this had increased to 11 institutions of higher education offering 14 Masters programs in public health. Currently, there are at least 17 Master of Public Health courses in Australia. This growth has occurred in conjunction with the identification of the importance of public health problems in the nation's health agenda, as discussed in a previous section. Of the annual intake of students into these degrees, at least half are usually medical graduates, with the remainder coming from allied health and nursing backgrounds. Very few psychologists, however, have so far enrolled in such degrees in this country.

Most of these degrees offer programs in health promotion and behavioural medicine aimed at integrating behavioural and public health science perspectives and methodologies. In one such Masters program at the University of Sydney all students undertake a half year course in health promotion and disease prevention, which is followed by eight more specialised optional courses in the second half of the year. These more specialised courses include "Health Promotion Theory," "Research Methods and Health Indices," "Behavioural Epidemiology," "Health Promotion in Clinical Settings," and "Community Development and Public Policy."

DISCUSSION

Health psychology in Australia can be seen to have developed out of a strong social-activist emphasis among psychologists involved in work on behaviour modification and therapy, out of work often carried on by psychologists working with psychiatry and other medical specialties, and out of the stimulus provided by some researchers working within university departments of psychology. More recent developments in public health and primary prevention of disease have provided new opportunities for health psychology research in this country (see Taylor and Owen, 1989). There are now many active and productive health psychology researchers; however, the undergraduate and graduate training of psychologists does not yet have any strong health emphasis, except in a few centres.

The Australian Psychological Society has established a working party on health psychology, and it seems likely that recommendations about the education of psychologists will flow from that initiative. However, this may take some time, and will probably occur in graduate, rather than undergraduate, psychology curricula. Furthermore, it seems likely that health psychology will develop most rapidly and extensively in interdisciplinary programs for a range of health professions, rather than exclusively from within the discipline of psychology itself. Behavioural medicine and health promotion are interdisciplinary areas which are providing strong leadership, opportunities for employment and relevant graduate training, and are fostering research in health psychology in Australia. The discipline of Psychology itself is lagging behind somewhat at present, but recent activities of psychologists and the Australian Psychological Society are likely to result in some strong initiatives from within the discipline in the near future.

References

Best, J. A. and Proctor, S. (1988). Behavioural medicine training from a public health perspective. *Annals of Behavioural Medicine* **10**, 19–22.

Better Health Commission (1986) *Looking forward to better health (Vol. 1–Vol 3).* Canberra: AGPS.

Birrell, P. and Lovibond, S. (1986). Historical and conceptual aspects. In King, N. J. and Remenyi, A. *Health care: A behavioural approach.* Sydney: Grune and Stratton.

Borland, R., Owen, N, Chapman, S. and Hill, D. (in press). Acceptance of workplace bans on smoking in Commonwealth Government offices. *Medical Journal of Australia.*

Califano, J. A. (1979). *Healthy people: The Surgeon General's Report on health promotion and disease prevention.* Washington, D.C.: U.S. Government Printing Office.

Dadds, M. R. (1988). Behaviour modification in Australia: A quantitative review of the last decade *Behaviour Change.* 5, 147–153.

Feletti, G., Firman, D. and Sanson-Fisher, R. (1986). Patient satisfaction with primary-care consultations. *Journal of Behavioural Medicine,* **9**, 389–400.

Groth-Marnat, G. (1988). A survey of the current and future directors of professional psychology in acute general hospitals in Australia. *Australian Psychologists,* **23**, 127–135.

Hetzel, B. S. and McMichael, A. J. (1987). *The LS factor.* Melbourne: Penguin.

Hill, D. J. (1988). Australian patterns of tobacco smoking in 1986. *Medical Journal of Australia,* **149**, 6–12.

Innes, J. M. and Owen, N. (1980). Social and behavioural dimensions of community health: An introductory course on psychology in health-care settings. *Australian Psychologist,* **15**, 169–180.

King, N. J. and Remenyi, A. (Eds) (1986). *Health care: A behavioural approach.* Sydney: Grune and Stratton.

Lovibond, S. H., Birrell, P. C. and Langeluddecke, P. (1986). Changing coronary heart disease risk factor status: The effects of three behavioral programs. *Journal of Behavioral Medicine,* **9**, 415–438.

Martin, P. R. (1986). Headaches. In N. J. King and A. Remenyi (Eds.) *Health care: A behavioural approach* (pp 145–158) Sydney: Grune and Stratton.

Martin, P. R. (1988). The teaching of health psychology in Australia. *Health Psychology Update,* **2** 3–6.

Millard, R. J. and Oldenburg, B. (1983) The symptomatic, urodynamic and psychological results of bladder re-education programmes. *Journal of Urology,* **130**, 715–720.

Oldenburg, B. and Byrne, D. G. (1986). Psychological management in the secondary prevention of myocardial infarction. In N. J. King and A. Remenyi (Eds.) *Health care: A behavioural approach.* Sydney: Grune and Stratton.

Oldenburg, B., Perkins, R J. and Andrews, G. (1985). A controlled trial of psychological intervention in myocardial infarction. *Journal of Consulting and Clinical Psychology,* **53**, 852–859.

Owen, N. and Dwyer, T. (1988). Approaches to promoting more widespread participation in physical activity. *Community Health Studies,* **12**, 339–347.

Owen, N. and Halford, W. K. (1988). Psychology, public health and cigarette smoking. *Australian Psychologist,* **23**, 137–152.

Owen, N. and Lee, C. (1986). Towards more rigorous evaluation of health promotion programmes. *Australian Psychologist,* **21**, 79–91.

Ross, M. W. (1988). Prevalence of risk factors for AIDS infection in the Australian population. *Medical Journal of Australia,* **149**, 362–365.

Sanson-Fisher, R. (1984). *Health behaviour research in Australia. New Zealand and Papua New Guinea: An overview.* Geneva: World Health Organization.

Sanson-Fisher, R. (1984). Commentary: Behavioural science and its relation to medicine—a need for positive action. *Community Health Studies,* **9**, 275–283.

Sax, S. (1984). *A strife of interests.* Sydney: Allen and Unwin.

Sheppard, J. L. (1982–1987). *Advances in Behavioural Medicine.* (Volume 1–Volume 4). Sydney: Cumberland College of Health Sciences.

Taylor, C. B. and Owen, N. (1989). Behavioural medicine: Research and development in disease prevention. *Behaviour Change,* **6**, 3–11.

Tiller, J. W. and Martin, P. R. (Eds.) (1980). *Proceedings of the Geigy Psychiatric Symposium on Behavioural Medicine.* Sydney: Ciba–Geigy.

Wilson, P. H. (1987). In memory of Robin Winkler: His contribution to behaviour modification in Australia. *Behaviour Change,* **4**, 3–10.

Winefield, H. R. and Peay, M. Y. (1980). *Behavioural science in medicine.* London: Allen and Unwin/ Beaconsfield.

Winkler, R. C. (1974). Research into mental health practice using pseudopatients. *Medical Journal of Australia,* **2**, 399–403.

Winkler, R. C. (1976). New directions for behaviour modification in homosexuality, open education and behavioural economics. In P. W. Sheehan and K. D. White (eds), "Behaviour modification in Australia" *Australian Psychologist,* **11**, Monog. Suppt, No. 3, 70–84.

Winkler, R. C. and Krasner, L. (1987) A social history of behaviour modification in Australia. *Behaviour Change,* **4**, 11–25.

Yates, A. J. (1979). *Biofeedback and the modification of behavior*, New York: Plenum Press.

CHAPTER 5

HEALTH PSYCHOLOGY IN CHINESE SOCIETIES IN ASIA

FANNY M. CHEUNG

Department of Psychology
The Chinese University of Hong Kong, Shatin, N. T. Hong Kong

This account of health psychology in four Chinese societies begins by outlining some distinguishing aspects of health behaviour and health care in these societies where tradional Chinese and western medicine co-exist. The overview shows that the field is still in an early stage of development. As a profession it is not yet well established and is mostly an extension of clinical psychology in non-psychiatric settings. There are a small number of psychologists working in general health care settings, with a greater involvement in treatment than in prevention. Also there is a small but growing research base and some of this work is briefly described.

Health Psychology is a new field in Chinese societies where Psychology itself is a relatively new discipline and profession. Although the first psychology department was established at Beijing University back in 1920s, the Sino-Japanese War, the founding of the People's Republic of China in 1949 and especially the Cultural Revolution in the 1960s resulted in halts to its development. Departments of Psychology in the People's Republic of China were resumed in late 1970s. The first Psychology departments in Taiwan and in Hong Kong were founded in the late 1940s and the mid 1960s respectively. To date, Psychology is not yet offered from an independent major department in Singapore. However, there are psychologists teaching, practising, and doing research in medical settings in all four countries whose works reflect the range of interests in the area. The following overview identifies common themes in Chinese Health Psychology and highlights the subject areas undertaken by psychologists in China, Hong Kong, Singapore and Taiwan.

HEALTH CARE AND HEALTH BEHAVIOUR IN CHINESE SOCIETIES

In traditional Chinese medicine, a strong relationship between the body and the mind is emphasized. Illnesses are discussed in terms of the balance of the *Yin* and *Yang* forces and the five fundamental elements (metal, wood, water, fire, and earth) which interact in harmony with similar forces and elements in nature (Huangti, 1967). The body is regarded as a microcosm in symbolic resonance with the social macrocosm as well as with the cosmos (Porkert, 1974). Illnesses are attributed to three groups of aetiological factors: six seasonal influences (wind, heat, fire, cold, moisture, and dryness), seven strong emotions (joy, grief, fear, anger, love, hatred, and desire), and situational conditions (trauma, fatigue, irregular diet, and insects, etc.). Conceptions of illness are based on integrated and dialectical notions of the physical and ecumenical systems (Porkert, 1974). Descriptions of the traditional Chinese medical system may be found in a number of books and articles (e.g. Chin and Chin, 1969; Koran, 1972; Topley, 1970; Unschuld, 1985).

Despite the import of western medicine in the early twentieth century and its present dominance in the formal medical practice of all the Chinese societies in Asia, traditional Chinese medicine has remained a popular modality of treatment among patients. Lee (1980) surveyed a large sample of Chinese in Hong Kong and found that over half reported using secular Chinese medicine in addition to or in combination with modern western-style medicine for treating diseases or in strengthening constitution. The Chinese medical tradition was considered to be as good as or even better than western scientific medicine because of its emphasis on tonic care, cure of the causes of diseases rather than symptomatic treatment, and fewer side effects from its treatment. A common process of a patient's treatment episode is self-medication using Chinese and/or western home remedies, consultation with a western-style doctor, consultation with a traditional Chinese medical practitioner or herbalist, and then attendance at a western medical hospital.

The implication of the coexistence of traditional Chinese medicine and western-style medicine may be reflected in the manifestation of illnesses and the process of help-seeking among the Chinese. Utilization of indigenous healing resources prior to western-style psychiatric treatment by patients have been noted in Hong Kong (Cheung, Lau, and Wong, 1984) and in Taiwan (Wen, 1990). Cheung et al. reported that neurotic patients initially sought help successively from western-style practitioners and Chinese herbalists before eventually being attended by a psychiatrist, which may be delayed by up to 30 years. Similar patterns of help-seeking were found by Wen in his study of psychiatric patients treated in a Buddhist temple in Taiwan. Wen classified four groups of healing modalities which have been sought by chronic schizophrenic patients: the popular sector includes herbs, secret recipes, massage, Chinese- or western-style tonics and non-prescriptive drugs; the folk-healing sector includes shamanism, physiognomy, geomancy, temple worship, spirit calling; the traditional-professional sector includes traditional Chinese medicine, bonesetting, and acupuncture; the western professional sector includes general medical clinic, general hospital, and psychiatric clinic or hospital. The intertwined utilization of these modalities suggests that patients tend to take a global, multidimensional view of their illness experience as opposed to the biomedical model of western medicine which adopts a causative and logico-deductive approach from the practitioner's perspective (Engel, 1977).

The different orientations of the two medical systems may account for discrepancy in the interpretation of the Chinese patients' illness experience by western-trained practitioners. Early studies on the patterns of symptom manifestation among Chinese psychiatric patients have observed that they tend to somatize their psychological problems and delay psychiatric consultation (Kleinman, 1977; Tseng, 1975). Psychological distress is presented in the form of bodily symptoms which may be viewed as idioms of distress (Kleinman, 1980, 1986). The western-style general practitioner is usually the first medical professional approached by a patient under physical or psychological distress. To the patient, the experience of distress is often global and undifferentiated, which is consistent with the folk concepts of Chinese medicine. There is no deliberate distinction between the body and the psyche, nor is there a sophisticated understanding of the various specializations among the medical profession which separates the body and the psyche. The medical practitioner is expected to relieve his/her suffering which often includes somatic symptoms. The suffering from somatic symptoms is usually the immediate reason for seeking professional medical help.

Kleinman noted the dominance of somatic complaints among psychiatric patients in Taiwan and among neurasthenic patients in the People's Republic of China (Kleinman, 1977, 1980, 1986). This tendency to report somatic symptoms may be interpreted by a western-trained physician as a masking of affective features or as a maladaptive coping style. The early reports of the somatization tendency among Chinese is based on the assumption of an artificial dichotomy between somatization and psychologization. The dichotomy implies that since Chinese patients tend to present their psychological problems in somatic forms, they are unaware of their psychological distress or would suppress such feelings. Post hoc explanations have been offered attributing this tendency to various aspects of the Chinese culture (Cheung, 1982). These oversimplified analyses of the phenomenon have been disputed in a series of empirical studies in Hong Kong and in China.

By having a psychiatrist interview the medical patients attending a general medical clinic in urban Hong Kong, Lau, Cheung, and Waldmann (1981) found that depressive disorders may be diagnosed among 8–20% of the daily intake of patients. The initial complaints reported by these patients to the general practitioner included bodily symptoms, especially those related to the central nervous system, general ill health, the gastrointestinal system, and the gynecological system for women. Cheung, Lau, and Waldmann (1980–1981) further distinguished between the expression mode and the recognition mode of symptom manifestation. Although the patients reported somatic complaints to the medical practitioner initially, upon being asked directly, they admitted the presence of affective features including feelings of sadness, nervousness, restlessness, and suicidal ideation. The solicitation of psychological expression may depend on the sensitivity and interviewing skills of the attending physician.

At the same time, patients may selectively report their illness experience according to their perception of the nature of the consultation. Cheung and Lau (1982) showed that patients attending a general outpatient clinic, a psychiatric clinic, and a prison clinic would bring forth different reasons for consultation in accordance with the situational context. Patients at the general outpatient clinic reported mostly somatic symptoms, patients at the psychiatric clinic presented a combination of somatic and psychological symptoms, whereas patients at the prison clinic usually recounted the antecedent events which led to their incarceration without reporting any medical symptoms.

Detailed studies on patients' report and presentation of symptoms further showed that psychological and somatic symptoms are not usually exclusive but are often presented in combination. Cheung, Lau, and Wong (1984) found that psychiatric patients seen at psychiatric clinics used both psychological and somatic concepts to describe their initial and their present problems. Patients who conceptualized their initial problems in mixed terms approached medical professionals early on and reached psychiatric resources soonest (Cheung, 1987).

In Kleinman's (1982) study of neurasthenic patients in China, he found that headache was one of the chief complaints presented to the physician, followed by insomnia and dizziness. However, the psychological complaints of poor memory, anxiety, irritability and disturbing dreams were also reported. When directly asked, all of the patients admitted having some forms of dysphoria including feelings of depression, sadness; displeasure, unhappiness, and irritability.

Zheng, Xu, and Shen (1986) studied the styles of verbal expression of emotional and physical experiences among depressed patients and normal controls in China. They classified four categories of verbal expression styles: purely psychological (e.g. unhappy; fearful), purely somatic (e.g. heart beating, losing weight), neutral (including both psychological and somatic features, e.g. uncomfortable inside heart; cannot use my brain), and deficient expression style (in which the person is unable or unwilling to choose an expression). They found that with abstract emotional terms involving feeling states such as indecisiveness, self-pity, guilt, or helplessness, the Chinese tend to adopt the psychological style of expression. With the concrete emotional state of fear, the most common expression style was somatic. The neutral mode was adopted for the expression of anxiety, whereas both the somatic and the neutral modes may be used for the expression of depression. In the case of suicidal ideation, the deficient style was used as a form of denial or suppression. These styles of expression might be changed by or interact with the individual's perception of his/her psychological and physical experiences. However, the frequency of using the somatic style in expressing emotions was not related to the report of somatic symptoms on a symptom check list. The lack of direct relationship between styles of verbal expression and somatization in the form of symptom manifestation suggests that the latter involves a multidimensional model which includes the physical concomitants of the problem, psychological conceptualizations, perceived solutions, and actual availability of these solutions.

Kleinman (1986) broadened the concept of somatization among the Chinese from that of the manifestation of depression in bodily complaints and that of a pathway of medical help-seeking to include an anthropological perspective. In his more recent analysis of somatization, the phenomenon 'includes interpretive schema for making sense of life problems . . . , rhetorical devices for controlling local relationships by persuading others . . . to provide greater access to scarce resources and empower the somatizer . . . , and symbolic forms that constitute and express salient modesl of life in particular cultures' (p. 173). This sociocultural perspective may be extended to the understanding of the psychological process of help seeking.

A person's illness experience is first defined according to his/her own conceptual schema or those of the significant others. These conceptualizations are in turn shaped by personal history, social expectations, and cultural norms. Whether or when these illness experiences will be presented to the professional may depend on these conceptualizations.

Cheung, Lee, and Chan (1983) investigated how students conceptualize five common somatic and psychological problems and what they intend to do about the problems. Students generally did not seek any professional help when the problems were considered mild. When they did seek help, they tended to approach a medical practitioner even when the problem might not be attributed to somatic causes. The medical professional was the most familiar figure among the helping professions whereas mental health professionals were relatively unknown even to college students. As long as there were somatic symptoms associated with the problems, medical consultation would be considered a means to alleviate that aspect of the suffering especially when self-help means were no longer effective.

Most Chinese would go through a process of self-help or social support network prior to seeking professional help. If the distress was perceived to be purely psychological in nature, or mild in its degree of severity, then self-reliance would be adopted (Cheung, Lee, and Chan, 1983). Active coping methods (e.g. analyzing the problem, resetting goals, and working harder) and psychological endurance (e.g. telling oneself to be claim, to accept or to forget the problem, and to control one's thoughts) were commonly used among students. Similar patterns of coping with daily problems were identified by Hwang in Taiwan (1977; 1978; 1979). The most common strategies adopted by Taiwanese men were the more passive means of learning to live with their problems, or facing the problems and persevering. Only the younger age groups and those from higher social class were more likely to adopt the more active problem-solving approaches. These passive and resigned attitudes were also observed among lower class psychiatric patients in Hong Kong (Cheung, Lau, and Wong, 1984).

IMPLICATIONS FOR HEALTH PSYCHOLOGY

Although most of the studies on help-seeking and problem conceptualizations have been conducted with regard to mental health, the findings show that mental health and physical health services are closely linked in the mind of the patients. If problems are conceptualized as purely psychological in nature, the Chinese would prefer to seek help from their friends or family (Cheung, 1984). If the problems are defined as symptoms of an illness, they would generally go to a medical physician. Distinctions among medical and mental health specialties are made by the professionals themselves. Psychological services are relatively unknown to the public partly due to the limited scope of these services in Chinese societies in Asia, as well as a low level of public health education.

The dominant role played by the medical practitioner is confirmed by the help-seeking studies reported earlier. In the paths to treatment, the general practitioner may be compared to a roundabout where routes may converge and be redirected. When most travellers were unfamiliar with the direct route to recovery, the roundabout was the hub they would return to before embarking on alternative treatment paths.

The relevance of psychological services in general practice is apparent. Given the interplay of psychology and medical care among the Chinese, Health Psychology should, then, be an important field to develop. However, the present stage of its development in Chinese societies is still rudimentary. Most psychologists working in the medical settings are attached to departments of psychiatry. An independent discipline of Health Psychology is not well established in China, Hong Kong, Singapore, or Taiwan. The status of Health Psychology may be examined in terms of its separate identity as a professional specialty as well as its specialized areas of research.

HEALTH PSYCHOLOGY AS A PROFESSION

Professional careers relating Psychology to health services in most of these Chinese societies have been restricted to Clinical Psychology. Most of the Clinical Psychologists work in psychiatric settings, with a minority working in areas of developmental handicap, family services, or correctional services. Although Clinical Psychologists have traditionally been involved heavily in assessment, some have become more actively engaged in psychological treatment in recent years. Since Clinical Psychologists are mostly trained in western models of Psychology, the assessment and treatment methods are mainly borrowed or translated.

In the People's Republic of China, the resumption of Psychology in the late 1970s has witnessed a growing interest in western assessment techniques, with a proliferation of efforts to translate common psychological tests. The field of Clinical Psychology was originally called Medical Psychology and no postgraduate training was offered to train psychologists working in psychiatric settings. In recent years, training in Clinical Psychology has been established, but the lack of qualified trainers limited its scope and standard. A number of textbooks on Medical Psychology have been written by psychologists or psychiatrists, which may be modelled after western textbooks in the field (X.T. Li, 1985; Yan, 1982). Medical Psychology is defined in more generic terms and consists of branches including Abnormal Psychology, Clinical Psychology, Neuropsychology, Mental Handicap, Psychosomatic Medicine, Psychodiagnosis, Psychotherapy and Counselling, and Mental Health. Psychological problems in general hospitals are discussed especially in relations to surgical patients, intensive care unit patients, traumatic injury, chronic illness, oncology patients and organ transplant patients. The types of psychosomatic illnesses introduced in the textbooks include cardiovascular disorders, hypertension, asthma, ulcer, obesity, and pain. These textbooks are written as much for medical students as for psychology students. However, in actual practice, the number of psychologists working in medical settings is extremely small given the small number of psychology students graduating from one of the six university departments offering a major degree in Psychology. The extent of the work of psychologists in medical settings is mostly limited to psychiatry.

Hong Kong provides master degree level training in Clinical Psychology modelled after the British training courses, and this postgraduate professional training is the minimum level required of Clinical Psychologists working in the medical settings. The majority of these Clinical Psychologists work in the government's mental health services. Only a couple of the psychologists' positions in these settings are extended beyond the psychiatry department to include liaison consultation from other medical departments in a general hospital. The most frequent sources of referral for liaison work are from Departments of Pediatrics, Oncology, Orthopedic and Traumatic Injury, Surgery, and Medicine. Clinical Psychologists are also involved in the postgraduate training of psychiatrists as well as the teaching of behavioural science in undergraduate medical education. These positions in the Medical Faculty may be situated in the Department of Psychiatry or the Department of Community Medicine. The role of the Medical Psychologist in general medicine has been discussed by Lee and his associates (Lee, 1984; Sharp and Fielding, 1985). Despite the emphasis on professionalism and the general positive response for the liaison consultation, the small number of psychologists again limit their impact in the field of Health Psychology.

In Singapore, the teaching of Psychology is offered under the joint Department of Social Work and Psychology. The Department of Psychological Medicine in the Faculty of Medicine is primarily a department of psychiatry. There is no postgraduate training in Clinical Psychology. The practising Clinical Psychologists are mostly trained overseas while a few may not have had specialized professional training. Most practising Clinical Psychologists work in psychiatric settings and are concerned with assessment. The size of the psychological community in Singapore is the smallest among the four Chinese societies.

Psychology in Taiwan has been better established, with undergraduate major programmes as well as postgraduate training programmes. Professions in Clinical Psychology are served by graduates of a first degree in Psychology in addition to those with postgraduate degrees. Psychologists work in the mental health services as well as in public health, where the issues studied in Health Psychology are more similar to those investigated in other western countries. Although translated psychological tests were commonly used in the early days, more locally developed Chinese tests have been constructed in recent years. However, the interest in Health Psychology outside of mental health is relatively new, and its impact on health services is not yet widespread.

RESEARCH IN HEALTH PSYCHOLOGY

Psychological research is mostly conducted by psychologists working in academic settings in all four Chinese societies, whereas funding and resources for research in applied settings are much more restricted. The number of researchers in Health Psychology is therefore very small. Some of the studies are conducted by other medical professionals who are interested in psychological factors in their particular areas of concern.

Medical Psychology in the People's Republic of China has adopted an emphasis on the physiological approach which was deemed to be more 'scientific'. Before the Cultural Revolution in the 1960s, a strong tradition of Pavlovian experimental psychology has directed the focus of research to the physical correlates of mental illness, especially schizophrenia, neurasthenia, mental retardation, and hyperkinesis (Chin and Chin, 1969). There was a strong interest in neurasthenia as a psychosomatic illness (Son, 1962; Wang and Lee, 1960). The opening of China to western psychology in the late 1970s has broadened the interest of Medical Psychology to include what was considered behavioural medicine and preventive medicine in the U.S. (Li, 1985).

A review of the major psychology and medical journals in China in the past decade show that the emphases of research in the area remained in the physiological and psychophysiological aspects of illness. For example, there were studies on the psychophysiological arousal and habituation of cardiovascular patients (Zhang, Chen, Liu and Chen, 1983), GSR and biofeedback training in controlling test anxiety (Sun, Zhao, Xia, Ren, Yan, Yang, Kao, and Wang, 1986), physiological responses to stress including heart rate, blood pressure, and immunological responses (Yang, Lin, Wang, Song, and Zhu, 1989), sleep and mental functions including memory, personality and adjustment (Fang, 1984; D.M. Li, 1985, 1987). A number of reports involved clinical case studies such as psychological profiles of kidney malfunctioning (Liu, Liu, Mei, Xu, Tchu, Sun, Zhiang, Chen, and Chen, 1989), psychological and physiological characteristics of patients with congenital insensitivity to pain (Xu, Wu, Sun, Zhang, Yan, and Du, 1984), and the developmental status and the causes of blindness among blind students (Lu, Yeh, Li, Zhang, Niu, and Zhang, 1987). Stress and life events have also been studied in relations to neurosis (Zheng and Young, 1983). Epidemiological studies such as the correlates of the prevalence of illness and utilization of medical care in a district of Beijing (Chen, Xu, Xu, and Sun, 1987) were also found. Recent interests in traditional forms of relaxation and exercises such as Qigong has resulted in a surge of studies claiming success in the treatment of hypertension, neurasthenia, psychosomatic disorders, and cancer, as well as in improving emotional stability and intelligence (Qian, 1990; Wang, 1989, 1990). Some of the authors of these studies were psychologists whereas many of the others were psychiatrists or physicians.

In Hong Kong, a number of Clinical Psychologists working closely with the medical school have studied patient compliance (Lee and Hung, 1983), adherence to cardiac rehabilitation (Fielding, 1987, 1989), psychological reactions of hand injury patients (Lee, Ho, Tsang, Cheng, Leung, Cheng and Lieh-Mak, 1985; Tsoi, Leung, and Chow, 1982; Tsoi, Leung, Chow, and Lee, 1985), and perceptions of children's distress and illness behaviours (Fielding and Tam, 1989). Women's health issues have also been studied in a psychological perspective by psychologists (Tsoi, 1985; Tsoi and Ho, 1984; Tsoi, Ho, and Poon, 1984; Tsoi, Poon and Ho, 1983) as well as by other medical professionals such as on the psychological reactions to gynaecological surgery (Alagaratnam and Kung, 1985; Tang, 1985a, 1985b), the needs and emotional states of women with carcinoma of the ovary or with gestational trophoblastic disease (Ngan and Tang 1984, 1986), or on sexual functioning following cancer treatment (O'Hoy and Tang, 1984; Ngan and Tang, 1988). An increasing interest in Health Psychology research has been reflected in the master theses submitted by Clinical Psychology trainees in recent years which include topics beyond that of mental illness.

The number of studies related to Health Psychology found in Singapore was even smaller. Since there were few psychologists working closely with the medical profession, and few mental health professionals working on non-psychiatric topics, only a couple of studies on stress associated with hospitalization or on psychological aspects of patients with chronic renal failure have been conducted by a Clinical Psychologist who has since left Singapore (Boey, 1984, 1988).

Influenced by the pioneering epidemiological studies on psychiatric illness in Taiwan, the earlier studies conducted by psychologists have focussed on mental health issues among normal people such as mental health problems among high school and college students (Ko, 1975, 1976; Ko, Yang, Cheng, and Yang-Lee, 1975; Miao, 1976; Yang, 1980; Yeh, Chu, Ko, Lin, and Lee, 1972). Clinical Psychologists and Social Psychologists have collaborated in studies related to coping with urban crowding (Hwang, 1979), stressful life events (Chang, Wu, and Hwu, 1985; Huang, Hwang, and Ko, 1983; Yeh, Ko, and Hwang, 1981) as well as stress and coping (Hwang, 1978, 1981; Ko, 1980). More recent studies have included public health topics such as stress and coping among mastectomy patients (Chang, Huang, and Lin, 1988) and drug abuse among adolescents (Chang, Hwang, Cheng, Wu, Lin and Yau, 1989).

DISCUSSION AND CONCLUSION

This brief overview of Health Psychology in four Chinese societies in Asia shows that the field is still in its early stage of development. As a profession, Health Psychology is not well established and is mostly an extension of conventional Clinical Psychology into nonpsychiatric consultation. The number of psychologists working in general health care settings is small, and their work is more concerned with treatment and consultation than with prevention and health care planning.

In terms of research, only some of the recent studies are extending their topics beyond mental health. Except for the studies in Hong Kong and Singapore, most of the other papers were written in the Chinese language. Until recent years, more of the studies addressing clinical aspects of mental or physical illness were found among the studies in Hong Kong. Studies in China emphasized the physiological aspects of illness (Ho, Spinks, and Yeung, 1989). Most of these studies are descriptive in nature. Some have covered psychological factors related to a range of physical and psychosomatic disorders, reflecting an orientation in Medical Psychology. There is still a strong link to traditional concerns in psychiatry. Little has been written in terms of primary prevention and health behaviour. The surge of interest in traditional forms of relaxation and exercise in recent years such as Qigong and Taichi will bring the realm of research more into prevention and health promotion.

The development of the field of Health Psychology will be affected by shortage of professional personnel and the insufficient recognition for the role of Psychology in medicine. With the small number of psychologists in general, and Clinical Psychologists in particular, an independent profession of Health Psychology is unlikely to be established in the near future. However, there is a growing interest among Clinical Psychologists to work beyond a psychiatric setting, and their services are beginning to be recognized by other medical professionals. Health Psychology is also included in the curriculum of some of the existing Clinical Psychology training programmes.

A fruitful direction for building up a theoretical framework in Health Psychology in Chinese societies lies in the integration of the mind and the body in the traditional Chinese concept of health. The folk concepts of Chinese medicine contains heavy emphasis on tonic care and prevention, which extend beyond the disease model. The existing literature on the nature of problem conceptualization, mode of distress expression, sources of social support, and patterns of formal help-seeking consists of studies conducted in the context of mental health. These same cultural concepts affect the general health behaviours of Chinese people across different social and political systems.

A typical illustration of these issues may be found in the study of neurasthenia. Neurasthenia is presented by Chinese patients as a form of physical illness in general practice. Even in the early days of political turmoils in the People's Republic of China, neurasthenia was a safe area of study for psychosomatic medicine (Cheung, 1989). While it often serves as an euphemism for mental illness, it conveys other tacit problems including family, work and political crises (Kleinman, 1986, 1988). A special journal volume was edited by Lin (1989) on neurasthenia among the Chinese.

Kleinman (1988) has proposed a framework for understanding the meanings of illness in terms of symptom, cultural significance, and life world. The individual's physical and psychological experience interacts with his/her environment and life trajectory in a dialectical manner. The major steps in the 'medical psychotherapeutic process' involves the tasks of a mini-ethnographic description to understand the illness experience from the patient's social and cultural perspective, the interpretation of the life history in the patient's personal context of illness, and the elicitation and negotiation of the patient's and the physician's explanatory models.

This psycho-social-cultural approach will provide a useful theoretical framework to understand health and health-seeking behaviour beyond the illness experience, an important area of concern in Health Psychology among Chinese as well as across cultures.

References

Alagaratnam, T.T. and Kung, N.Y.T. (1985). The psychosocial sequelae of mastectomy in Chinese females. *Journal of the Hong Kong Psychiatric Association, 5,* 39–42.
Boey, K.W. (1984). A factor analysis of psychological reaction in patients undergoing haemodialysis. *Asian Medical Journal, 27,* 456–463.
Boey, K.W. (1988). The measurement of stress associated with hospitalization. *Singapore Medical Journal, 29,* 586–588.
Chan, D.W. and Chan-Ho, M.W. (1983). Stressful life events: overview and lessons from a Chinese context. *Journal of the Hong Kong Psychiatric Association, 3,* 3–7.
Chan, D.W., Chan, T.S.C., and Chan-Ho, M.W. (1984). Occurrence and co-occurrence of stressful life events in a Chinese context. *International Journal of Psychosomatics, 31,* 3–10.
Chang, C., Huang, M.G., and Lin, H.C. (1988). [Preliminary study on stressor and coping of mastectomy patients]. *Journal of National Public Health Association, 8,* 109–124. (In Chinese.)
Chang, C., Hwang, W.H., Cheng, M.K., Wu, S.C., Lin, H.C., and Yau, B.R. (1989). [Survey of substance abuse among adolescents]. *Public Health, 15,* 388–402. (In Chinese.)
Chang, L.Y., Wu, E.C., and Hwu, H.G. (1985). [The concept and measurement of life stress]. *Chinese Journal of Mental Health, 2,* 137–151. (In Chinese.)
Chen, Y.D., Xu, L.F., Xu., P.F., and Shun, H.K. (1987). [Determinants analysis of inhabitant's prevalence of illness and seek medical care in Xi-cheng district of Beijing City]. *Chinese Journal of Preventive Medicine, 21,* 268–2721. (In Chinese.)
Cheung, F.M. (1982). Psychological symptoms among Chinese in urban Hong Kong. *Social Science and Medicine, 16,* 1339–1344.
Cheung, F.M. (1984). Preference in help-seeking among Chinese students. *Culture, Medicine and Psychiatry, 8,* 371–380.
Cheung, F.M. (1987). Conceptualization of psychiatric illness and help-seeking behavior among Chinese. *Culture, Medicine and Psychiatry, 11,* 97–106.
Cheung, F.M. (1989). The indigenization of neurasthenia in Hong Kong. *Culture, Medicine, and Psychiatry, 13,*
Cheung, F.M. and Lau, B. (1982). Situational variations in help-seeking behavior among Chinese patients. *Comprehensive Psychiatry, 23,* 252–262.
Cheung, F.M., Lau, B.W.K., and Waldmann, E. (1980–81). Somatization among Chinese depressives in general practice. *International Journal of Psychiatry in Medicine, 10,* 361–374.
Cheung, F.M., Lau, B.W.K., and Wong, S.W. (1984). Paths to psychiatric care in Hong Kong. *Culture, Medicine and Psychiatry, 8,* 207–228.
Cheung, F.M. Lee, S.Y., and Chan, Y.Y. (1983). Variations in problem conceptualizations and intended solutions among Hong Kong students. *Culture, Medicine and Psychiatry, 7,* 263–278.
Chin, R. and Chin, A.L.S. (1969). *Psychological research in Communist China: 1949–1966.* Cambridge, MA: MIT Press.
Engel, G. (1977). The need for a new medical model: a challenge for biomedicine. *Science, 196,* 129–136.
Fang, J.D. (1984). [The physiological basis of the interaction between sleep and memory]. *Acta Psychologica Sinica,* No. 16, 223–230. (In Chinese.)
Fielding, R. (1987). Patients' beliefs regarding the causes of myocardial infarction: implications for information giving and compliance. *Patient Education and Counseling, 9,* 121–134.
Fielding, R. (1989). A note on early indicators of non-adherence to a cardiac rehabilitation programme. *British Journal of Medical Psychology, 62,* 97–101.
Fielding, R. and Tam, F.S.H. (1989). Role and context in the perception of distress. *Bulletin of the Hong Kong Psychological Society, 22/23,* 29–45.
Ho, D.Y.F., Spinks, J.A., and Yeung, C.S.H. (eds.) (1989). *Chinese patterns of behavior: a sourcebook of psychological and psychiatric studies.* New York: Praeger.
Huang, H.C., Hwang, K.K., and Ko, Y.H. (1983). [Life stress, attribution style, social support and depression among university students]. *Acta Psychologica Taiwanica, 25,* 31–47. (In Chinese.)
Huangti (author unknown) (1967). *Huangti neijing suwen* [The Yellow Emperor's classic of internal medicine, plain questions]. Reprinted from *Guang Shu* copy of the Qing Dynasty. Collection of *Gujin Yitung Zhengmai,* Vol. 2. Taipei: Yiwen.
Hwang, K.K. (1977). The patterns of coping strategies in a Chinese society. *Acta Psychologica Taiwanica, 19,* 61–73.
Hwang, K.K. (1978). The dynamic processes of coping with interpersonal conflicts in a Chinese society. *Proceedings of the National Science Council, 2,* 198–208.

Hwang, K.K. (1979). Coping with residential crowding in a Chinese urban society: the interplay of high-density dwelling and interpersonal values. *Acta Psychologica Taiwanica, 21,* 117–133.
Hwang, K.K. (1981). [Perception of life events: the application of non-metric multidimensional scaling]. *Acta Psychologica Taiwanica, 22,* 22–32. (In Chinese.)
Kleinman, A.M. (1977). Depression, somatization and the "new cross-cultural psychiatry". *Social Science and Medicine, 11,* 3–10.
Kleinman, A.M. (1980). *Patients and healers in the context of culture.* Berkeley, CA: University of California Press.
Kleinman, A.M. (1986). *Social origins of distress and disease: depression, neurasthenia, and pain in modern China.* New Haven: Yale University Press.
Kleinman, A.M. (1988). *The illness narratives: suffering, healing, and the human condition.* New York: Basic Books.
Ko. Y.H. (1976). The mental health of junior and senior high school boys. *Acta Psychologica Taiwanica, 18,* 37–52.
Ko, Y.H. (1980). *Mental Health, Vol. 1 – Theory.* Taipei: Tai Yang Publishers. (In Chinese.)
Koran, L.M. (1972). Psychiatry in mainland China: history and recent status. *American Journal of Psychiatry, 128,* 84–92.
Ko, Y.H., Yang, K.S., Cheng, H.H. and Yang-Lee, P.H. (1975). [The relationship between school environment and college student mental health]. *Bulletin of the Institute of Ethnology,* No. 39, 125–149. (In Chinese.)
Lau, B.W.K., Cheung, F.M., and Waldmann, E. (1981). Morbidity of depression illness in general practice. *Asian Medical Journal, 24,* 518–527.
Lee, P.W.H. (1984). Medical psychology: selective review and projection in Hong Kong. *Hong Kong Psychological Society Bulletin,* No. 13, 7–15.
Lee, P.W.H., Ho, E.S.Y., Tsang, A.K.T., Cheng, J.C.Y., Leung, P.C., Cheng, Y.H., and Lieh-Mak, F. (1985). Psychosocial adjustment of victims of occupational hand injuries. *Social Science and Medicine, 20,* 493–497.
Lee, P.W.H. and Hung, B.K.M. (1983). Understanding and improving patient compliance. *Hong Kong Practitioner, 5,* 553–560.
Lee, P.W.H., Sharp, I.J., and Fielding, R. (1985). The taming of the devil, the psychologist in the medical setting. *Hong Kong Psychological Society Bulletin,* No. 14, 78–83.
Lee, R.P.L. (1980). Perception and uses of Chinese medicine among the Chinese in Hong Kong. *Culture, Medicine and Psychiatry, 4,* 345–375.
Li, D.M. (1985). [A study on the relationship between sleep quality and some psychological functions of college students]. *Acta Psychologica Sinica,* 418–421.
Li, D.M. (1987). [A study on the relationship between sleep and mind health]. *Acta Psychologica Sinica,* 92–99.
Lin, T.Y. (1989). Neurasthenia in Asian Cultures. Special issue of *Culture Medicine and Psychiatry,* 13.
Liu, C.Z., Liu, X.H., Mei, Z.Y., Xu, K.Z. Tchu, J.L., Sun, T.C., Zhiang, H.L., Chen, D.R., and Chen, Y.G. (1989). [Depressive states among 18 cases of chronic kidney failure patients undergoing dialysis]. *Chinese Journal of Neurology and Psychiatry,* 22, 168–170. (In Chinese.)
Lu, Z.Z., Yeh, G.J., Li, Z.Y., Zhang, Y.L., Niu, W.Y., Zhang, Y.N. (1987). [An investigation on the developmental status and the causes of blindness of blind students]. *Chinese Journal of Preventive Medicine, 21,* 279–282. (In Chinese.)
Miao, E. (1976). An exploratory study on college freshmen mental health status. *Acta Psychologica Taiwanica, 18,* 129–147.
Ngan, Y.S. and Tang, G.W.K. (1984). Needs and emotional states in cancer patients: a study of 21 Chinese women with carcinoma of the ovary. *Journal of Psychosomatic Obstetrics and Gynaecology, 3,* 223–231.
Ngan, H.Y.S. and Tang, G.W.K. (1986). Psychosocial aspects of gestatinal trophoblastic disease in Chinese residents of Hong Kong. *Journal of Reproductive Medicine, 31,* 173–178.
Ngan, H.Y.S. and Tang, G.W.K. (1988). Further study of sexual functioning following treatment of carcinoma of the cervix on Chinese patients. *Journal of Psychosomatic Obstetrics and Gynaecology, 9,* 117–129.
O'Hoy, K.M. and Tang, G.W.K. (1985). Sexual function following treatment for carcinoma of cervix. *Journal of Psychosomatic Obstetrics and Gynaecology, 4,* 51–58.
Porkert, M. (1974). *The theoretical foundations of Chinese medicine: systems of correspondence.* Cambridge, MA: MIT Press.
Qian, M.Y. and Chen, J.G. (1990). Chinese traditional relaxation techniques and their effectiveness. Paper presented at the 22nd International Congress of Applied Psychology, Kyoto, Japan, July 22–27.

Son, W.C. (1962). [Some differences of the functional states of cerebral cortex in patients of neurasthenia, hypertension and peptic ulcer]. *Acta Psychologica Sinica,* No. 3, 241–247. (In Chinese.)
Sun, Z.X., Zhao, J.C., Xia, M.L., Ren, R.Z., Yan, H.J., Yang, L.L., Kao, X., and Wang, S.Z. (1986). [A comparative study on the effectiveness of GSR biofeedback and self-training on the control of test anxiety]. *Acta Psychologica Sinica,* 196–201. (In Chinese.)
Tang, G.W.K. (1985a). Emotional reactions to gynaecological surgery. *Hong Kong Psychological Society Bulletin,* No. 14, 5–7.
Tang, G.W.K. (1985b). Reactions to emergency hysterectomy. *Obstetrics and Gynecology, 65,* 206–210.
Topley, M. (1970). *Chinese traditional ideas and the treatment of disease: two examples from Hong Kong.* Hong Kong: Centre of Asian Studies Reprint Series no. 24, University of Hong Kong.
Tseng, W.S. (1975). The nature of somatic complaints among psychiatric patients: the Chinese case. *Comprehensive Psychiatry, 16,* 237–245.
Tsoi, M. (1985). Psychological contributions to understanding gynaecological problems. *Hong Kong Psychological Society Bulletin,* No. 14, 9–16.
Tsoi, M.M. and Ho, P.C. (1984). Psychological factors related to adjustment after tubal ligation. *Journal of Reproductive and Infant Psychology, 2,* 1–6.
Tsoi, M.M., Ho, P.C. and Poon, R.S. (1984). Preoperation indicators and post-hysterectomy outcome. *British Journal of Clinical Psychology, 23,* 151–152.
Tsoi, M.M., Leung, P.W.L., and Chow, S.P. (1982). Psychological reactions to hand injuries among semi-skilled Chinese workers. *Annals of the Academy of Medicine of Singapore, 11,* 214–217.
Tsoi, M.M., Leung, P.W.L., Chow, S.P., and Lee, P.C. (1985). Short-term reactions to hand injury caused by industrial accidents. *Journal of Hong Kong Psychiatric Association, 5,* 26–30.
Tsoi, M.M., Poon, R.S., and Ho, P.C. (1983). Knowledge about reproductive organs in Chinese women: some overlooked "common sense". *Journal of Psychosomatic Obstetrics and Gynaecology, 2,* 70–75.
Unschuld, P. (1985). *Medicine in China: a history of ideas,* Berkely, CA: University of California Press.
Wang, J.S. (1989) [*Chinese Qigong psychology*]. Beijing: Chinese Social Science Press. (In Chinese.)
Wang, J.S. (1990). Psychological study of Qigong. Paper presented at the 22nd International Congress of Applied Psychology, Kyoto, Japan, July 22–27.
Wang, J.S. and Lee, H.T. (1960). [Preliminary study of the etiology of neurasthenia]. *Acta Psychologica Sinica,* No. 1, 46–53. (In Chinese.)
Wen, J.K. (1990). The Hall of Dragon metamorphoses: a unique, indigenous asylum for chronic mental patients in Taiwan. *Culture, Medicine and Psychiatry, 14,* 1–19.
Xu, S.L., Wu, Z.Y., Sun, C.H., Y., X.W., Du, T.L., and Yang, Z.L. (1984). [The psychological and physiological characteristics of two patients with congenital insensitivity to pain. I. Emotional characteristics]. *Acta Psychologica Sinica,* 289–297. (In Chinese.)
Wong, J.W.P., Lau, L.S.Y., and Wong, V. (1984). Work stress among office workers in Hong Kong. *Hong Kong Journal of Mental Health, 13,* 66–73.
Yan, H.J. (ed.) (1982). *[Introduction to medical psychology]. Shangai: Shanghai Science and Technology Press. (In Chinese.)*
Yang, J., Lin, B.C., Wang, C.H., Song, C.Y., and Zhu, E.L. (1989). [The influence of psychological stress on blood pressure, heart rate, breathing, and immunological responses]. Acta Psychologica Sinica, 191–193. (In Chinese.)
Yeh, E.K., Chu, H.M., Ko, Y.H., Lin, T.Y., and Lee, S.P. (1972). [Student mental health: an epidemiological study in Taiwan]. *Acta Psychologica Taiwanica, 14,* 1–25. (In Chinese.)
Yeh, M.H., Ko, Y.H., and Hwang, K.K. (1981). [Life stress and mental health]. *Bulletin of the Institute of Ethnology.* (Academia Sinica), No. 52, 173–210. (In Chinese.)
Zhang, B.Y., Chen, Z.G., Liu, J., and Chen, K.Z. (1983). [A study on the psychosomatic reactions of cardiovascular patients: I. Arousal level and habitual orientation]. *Acta Psychologica Sinica,* 205–209. (In Chinese.)
Zheng, Y.P., Xu, L.Y., and Shen, Q.J. (1986). Styles of verbal expression of emotional and physical experiences: study of depressed patients and normal controls in China. *Culture, Medicine and Psychiatry, 10,* 231–243.
Zheng, Y.P. and Young, D. (1983). [The relationship of life event change and stress to neurosis]. *Chinese Journal of Neurology and Psychiatry, 9,* 65–68. (In Chinese.)

CHAPTER 6

CUBAN HEALTH PSYCHOLOGY: A PRIORITY IS THE PRIMARY HEALTH CARE SYSTEM

SØLVI KRISTIANSEN and KERSTIN SØDERSTRØM

Larkollen Inpatient Treatment Home for Adolescents, 1560 Larkollen, Norway

Cuban health psychology has experienced a great expansion during the last 25 years, both in the number of psychologists and in range of activities in the field. Today, psychologists are integrated at all levels of the national health system, an achievement which is particularly interesting in that Cuba is a developing country. In a position isolated from trends in international psychology, Cuba has developed a role for psychologists within the field of health which is adapted to its situation as a poor and socialistic country. Priority is given to preventive and community-based psychology within primary health care facilities. Psychologists in primary health care serve a composite client-group, with high priority given to pregnant women and to children. The work of these psychologists covers a wide range of health problems—physical as well as mental—and focuses upon individuals as bio-psycho-social units. Their responsibilities include health promotion, disease prevention, consultation and treatment, rehabilitation, research and education. This report is based on a 2½ month long field study in Cuba, where Cuban health psychology, particularly as it relates to primary health care, was explored.

INTRODUCTION

During the last 25 years, the field of Cuban health psychology has experienced great expansion, both in the number of psychologists working in the field, and in its range of activities. After the 1959 revolution, the new health authorities quickly recognized the important role psychology and its methods could play in defeating the country's health problems. As a result, psychologists today are integrated into all levels of the Cuban health system, in both administration and clinical work (Garcia, 1980; Garcia-Averasturi, 1985).

During this process of change and expansion, Cuban psychologists have had very limited access to information concerning developments in international psychology (Marin, 1985). This is the case, partly as a result of the US blockade of Cuba, and partly as a consequence of Cuba's lack of international currency. In spite of its isolated position, we see Cuban health psychology as being in accord with the basic principles of health psychology, community psychology and general guidelines for health services laid out by the World Health Organization, as cited in Garcia (1985) and Kristiansen and Søderstrøm (1987).

Cuban health psychologists have worked hard to develop a professional role which is adapted to the needs, resources and ideals of Cuban society (Garcia-Averasturi, 1985). With this aim in mind, they have found traditional psychology, with its focus on individuals and on the testing and treatment of mental illness, to be quite limited. Cuba's focus has been on the country's main health problems which at the time of the revolution were typically poverty related diseases, and today are health problems such as cancer, coronary/heart diseases, and other lifestyle related diseases. Other health related problems of priority are mother and child health and family conflicts. A preventive and community-based psychology in primary health care facilities is considered to be the most effective strategy to fight these problems.

The Cuban concept of health psychology refers to all health related psychological activities performed by psychologists employed by the Cuban Ministry of Public Health, MINSAP.† This would include health planning, health promotion, disease prevention, research, education, consultation, psychological treatment and rehabilitation. The focus of this concept is on both physical and mental health, and stresses the interconnections betwen psychological, social and biological factors (Morales, 1987).

The aim of this paper is to provide an overview of the current status of Cuban health psychology as well as its development. Special focus here is put on activities in primary health care facilities. We find the Cuban experiences to be very relevant to the general debate on the role of health psychology in primary health care today. Also taking into consideration Cuba's position as a developing country, its programs are of particular interest as possible models for the role of psychology in other developing countries.

METHOD

This report is based on a 2½ month long field study in Cuba during the winter of 1986/87. It was organized as a cooperation between the University of Bergen, Norway, and the Cuban Ministry of Health (MINSAP). Data were gathered through interviews with psychologists working in both health administration and in clinical work; through MINSAP statistics; through written material; and through day-to-day observations made in three basic health care clinics, in Cuba called policlinics. Observations and statistical data have been limited to the capital city of Havana (Ciudad de la Habana) and to a neighbouring province (Provincia de la Habana). The methodological problems involved in such a cross-national study have been dealt with extensively in a previous report (Kristiansen and Søderstrøm, 1987), and will not be focused on in this report.

PSYCHOLOGY IN THE NATIONAL HEALTH SYSTEM

Before the 1959 revolution there were very few psychologists in Cuba, these having been educated either abroad or in small private universities. None of these psychologists worked in public hospitals, which at the time, were inadequate and few. Three years after the revolution, two institutes of psychology were established under the Faculties of Science, one in Havana and one in Santa Clara, and in 1977 these institutes became faculties. It was in 1966 that the Ministry of Public Health (MINSAP) employed some of the first psychologists graduated after the revolution. The first task of those employed was to develop a curricula in psychology for use by physicians. Two years later, the National Group of Psychology (Grupo Nacional de Psicologia) was established, marking Cuba's first step towards a hierarchical organizational structure in the field of psychology. By this time Cuba had achieved an

† Ministero de Salud Publica.

integrated national health system that reached throughout the island. Also a new concept of health care was emerging, with the emphasis on prevention. Health was considered as a social phenomenon and proper health care as a right of every Cuban citizen (Garcia, 1980).

The objective of the National Group of Psychology was to develop a preventive and community-oriented psychology in accordance with the general health philosophy of the country. They agreed that primary health care facilities were the best settings for this, and in 1969 the first psychologists were integrated into the basic units of primary health care, the policlinics.

In order to strengthen the psychosocial aspects of the health services further, a new group of health professionals—psychometricians—emerged in 1973. Psychometricians undergo three years of training, which then qualifies them to assist psychologists. Psychometricians perform psychological testing, lead group discussions and colect data used in research.

Today, health psychology has grown into quite an influential field within the Cuban health services. Figures from 1985 show there were 256 psychologists and approximately the same number of psychometricians working within the public health services in Havana (MINSAP, 1985). This means approximately one psychologist and one psychometrician for every 7750 inhabitants, with primary health care continuing to be a priority area.

All psychologists in MINSAP, regardless of area of specialization, are part of an organization with functions at three levels—national, provincial and regional. This organization is governed by a principle of normative centralization and administrative decentralization (Morales, 1984). On a national level is the National Group of Psychology which consists of representatives from various regions of the country, and of one leader. Until 1987, this leader position was full-time. Today, however, this is a part-time position under the office of MINSAP central administration. This group's tasks include consulting the central health administration on the psychosocial aspects of health, performing nation-wide assessments and research, setting standards and developing guidelines for the work of psychologists within the health services, and evaluating psychological healthcare activity around the country. On the provincial level (Cuba has 14 provinces) we find the Provincial Group of Psychology. This group performs tasks similar to that of the National Group, but adapted to the particular needs of the provinces. In Havana, the leader of the Provincial Group of Psychology is employed full-time under the provincial administration of MINSAP. At the regional level, a psychologist from one of the policlinics in the region is engaged for part-time administrative tasks.

Basic Ideas: Marxist–Leninism and "Integrated" Psychology

The basic ideology of Cuban society is Marxist–Leninism. Within the field of psychology, this means that people's lives are seen as very closely connected to both material and social factors. Further, this means that the professional psychologist is obliged to work in the service of the working-class. This ideological platform is, however, very general. In practice. Cuban psychology seems to be both theoretically and empirically open, relating to the situations and the problems of people's everyday lives, and trying to resolve them.

It seems important to focus upon how health psychology is connected to a more general ideology of health and health services in Cuba. In 1974, new guidelines for the health service were launched, with community medicine as the basic concept. Some of the principles emphasized were integrated medicine, teamwork and community participation. We will discuss the idea of integrated medicine in greater detail, and particularly the notion of integrated psychology.

The concept of integrated medicine is closely related to a health-field concept, in which the individual is seen as a "bio-psycho-social" unit. This then means health services are planned and performed bearing in mind the complexity of an individual's make-up. Also, this concept implies that health services are responsible for health promotive, preventive, curative and rehabilitative activities. And furthermore, target groups are viewed as encompassing individuals, families, environments and societies. This concept lies in opposition to a limited biological and curative approach to health and illness.

To psychology this concept of integration has been and is of major importance. Through the concept's implicit acceptance of the influence of psychological factors on health, it has promoted the position of psychologists within the national health system. Further, the idea of integration is an important guiding principle to Cuban health psychologists, both concerning their activities and their organization. The Cubans don't want to limit health psychology to specific health problems, e.g., physical diseases, but include psychological aspects of different areas crucial to the public health. Francisco Morales, the leader of the Provincial Group of Psychology in Havana, says "Health psychology must work in different areas, from personality development to the promotion of a healthier lifestyle, in an integrated context. Health and illness must be seen as a continuing process, and the human being must be treated as a psychosomatic unit. From this extensive point of view health psychology can work with areas that apparently are distinct, but which are unified through a criterium of integation" (Morales, 1987, p. 8). This does not imply that there is no room for specialisation, but that integrated thinking must be used to guide the psychology services within the whole of the health services.

From this general platform the health psychologists give priority to those areas of health meant to be the most actual and important to their society. Today they focus particularly on mother–child health and the so called life style related diseases. Morales expressed in an interview that they find it important to face the needs of their society rather than follow the traditional fields of study in academic psychology. This statement also manifests the pragmatic orientation of Cuban health psychology, it has been and is more concerned with the resolution of practical problems than with theoretical discussions.

The principle of integration is also basic in the organization of the MINSAP psychologists. Though they are working in different specialization areas they are all organized in the Cuban Society of Psychology of Health. Also, in Havana there is a meeting for all MINSAP psychologists in the region once a month. Here they discuss academic and professional issues relevant to health psychology.

Primary Health Care

The basic facility of the Cuban primary health care system is the policlinic, each of which serves about 25,000–30,000 inhabitants.† Today there are one to three

† In the countryside there are also smaller medical services "Puestos Medicos" that serve 1000–2000 inhabitants.

psychologists employed in each of the policlinics in Havana. In 1985 it was decided to decentralize the health care system further, and a new plan involving family doctors was implemented. The family doctors work administratively through the policlinics, but live in the local neighbourhoods and serve about 150 families each. The idea began in a rural mountain area in eastern Cuba, but has developed to a national health plan through strong support from Fidel Castro. In January 1987, this plan was realized in 18 of Havana's 73 policlinics.

Whether or not an area has implemented the policy involving family doctors greatly influences psychologists' work routines. In areas without family doctors, contact between the policlinic's staff and their target groups is direct. In policlinics with family doctors, the medical specialist and psychologists visit the family doctors regularly; often having their first consultations with clients there. Frequently, psychologists and the family doctors also have consultations in which the psychologist advises the family doctor on the psychosocial aspects of health.

Psychologists in policlinics are generalists, their tasks include health education; consultation and therapy; and teaching and research. Visits to homes, schools, work-centers and to numerous local organizations are included in a Cuban psychologist's job. These visits are often performed together with other health personnel from the policlinic (physicians, social-workers etc.).

The guidelines for a psychologist's activity in a policlinic are formulated in plans by the National Group of Psychology. Today two plans exist, one for policlinics without family doctors and one for those with. Let us take a closer look at the latter plan, containing ten priority areas—all of which include concrete suggestions for action.

The ten priority areas for a psychologists's involvement are:

1) Education of family doctors and nurses in the psychosocial aspects of health.

2) Participation in programs for health promotion. Priority areas include smoking, encouraging physical activity, unhealthy eating habits, and alcohol abuse.

3) Work to reduce the number of unwanted pregnancies in the area† and to increase a community's knowledge of sexuality and reproduction.

4) Promote healthy relations and patterns of communication within family units.

5) Help those pregnant to cope emotionally, particularly those with high-risk pregnancies. This hopefully prevents complications during birth and promotes healthy development of the newborn.

6) Work to promote healthy development for children who are underweight at birth, and those who are at high risk—physically or socially.

7) Cooperate with institutions of education to promote the physical and psychological well-being of schoolchildren.

8) Contribute to healthy working conditions at local work-centers.

9) Help the chronically ill and their families to cope wth their particular situations.

10) Carry out assessments of the psychological aspects of the main health problems in the area.

This plan also includes norms for the amount of time spent on various areas. It is recommended that a psychologist spend about 27% of his/her work time with

† Unwanted pregnancy is recognized as one of the main health problems in Cuba.

pregnant women and their relations, 18% on health promotion work, 18% working with the chronically ill, 9% at schools, 9% in research and 18% in various other areas (MINSAP, 1986).

It is difficult to judge, due to the relatively short duration of our field study, just how closely the practice of health-psychology is in accordance with central guidelines. Our general impression is that practitioners are to a great degree fulfilling the central goals of the plan. The guidelines include however extensive detailing of tasks and target groups, which individual psychology departments in policlinics have no possibility of fulfilling. Our research noted that different policlinics had different priorities. Common to all the clinics we visited was the psychologists' practice of spending more than half of their time in clinical work, usually on individual and family consultations. Group therapy was also prevalent. Also, pregnant women and children represented high priority groups in all policlinics we visited. All pregnant women in each district are referred to the area psychologist from the general practitioner. The psychologist then interviews the women in order to assess the psychological and social risk factors of each. He/she also gives each woman (and her husband if he is attending) information about the psychological aspects of pregnancy and motherhood.

Health promotive and preventive work in schools, with local organizations and in work-centers was rather infrequent in our observation. Health education, however, was often a part of the individual and group consultations.

In interviews and conversations with psychologists, some expressed the desire to spend more time on health promotive and preventive work. The demand for direct psychological services is so great, however, that most of their time is occupied with this. It was added that they now want to educate family doctors in the psychosocial aspects of health; hoping that the physicians themselves could in the future manage some of the work they now are referring to the psychologists. This in turn would give psychologists more time for other aspects of their work.

A Milestone?

Fransicso Morales, head of the Provincial Group of Psychology in Havana, describes the present standing of health psychology in Cuba as a milestone in the field. They now have nearly 20 years of experience in the primary health care services, and during these years the country's health situation and needs have greatly changed. When the first psychologists graduated after the revolution and began to work in MINSAP, Cuba faced a health situation dominated by poverty-related diseases and with access to few material and technical resources. Today, the health situation is very similar to that of most industrialized countries with very well-organized health services reaching all of the population. The image that people have of psychologists is also much more positive, and the demand for psychological services in Cuban communities is great.

With the implementation of a plan utilizing family doctors, the whole organizational structure of the health services has changed, and the psychologist is constantly facing new challenges. It is therefore considered very important to continuously evaluate the cooperation and the psychologists' experiences, and discuss the coming developments in health psychology in this new context.

Other Activities

Though primary health care is a priority area, psychologists also work in secondary and tertiary health care, for example in psychiatry and in hospitals which care for people with physical problems. There does not as yet exist a national plan for this sort of work, but it continues to be a theme of discussion among psychologists in the health administration in Havana. We particularly want to note that departments of psychology are established in many children's hospitals, gynaecological–obstetrical hospitals and clinical surgical hospitals. Previously, psychologists worked in the psychiatric departments of hospitals, but now they have their own departments in cooperation with psychometricians. Their goals are to help clients and their families cope with the preparations for operations (or birth), the operation/birth itself, and for post-hospitalization life. Their aims include promoting healthy development for the ill; good psychosocial environments for the newborn, and preventing negative psychological and social effects of hospitalization.

Training in Health Psychology

Two Cuban universities, the University of Havana and the University of Santa Clara, have five year long specialization programs in psychology after secondary school. Both are based on a new generalist model of psychological study which has replaced the previous program which contained four areas of specialization: clinical psychology, social psychology, educational psychology and occupational psychology. After graduation, psychologists must take part in a three year service in rural areas of Cuba. This program insures the distribution of psychological services throughout the country. Although there are no organized graduate specialization programs for psychologists, seminars on special topics are often held by the MINSAP.

Confronted with the amount and variety of tasks covered in the field of health psychology, particularly in primary health care, a question emerges concerning how well the Cuban psychologists can be trained to perform these activities. In Palacios' 1986 survey concerning how well psychologists in primary health care facilities in Havana were trained to cope with the demands of their jobs, encouraging facts were discovered. She noted that the concordance between the psychologists' education and that of their job demands had become far better since the introduction of the generalist model of education. However, the training in areas such as those of health promotion and community-based activities is still considered insufficient. Palacios further concludes that there is a strong need for organized graduate specialization programs for health psychologists. In an interview with the Provincial Group of Psychology in Havana, members of the group expressed concern over this problem and informed us that future plans for possible graduate specialization programs were being discussed.

CONCLUSION

Cuban health psychology is today an integrated part of the Cuban health system, both on an administrative and a practical level. Cuba has developed a professional role for the psychologist within the health forces. This role focuses on preventive psychology and on the necessity of approaching human beings as bio-psyco-social units. Priority in the Cuban approach has been and is being given to primary health care facilities.

The impressive achievements in Cuban psychology, and particularly the development of their professional role within the national health care system, may provide an important contribution to a general debate on models for psychologists' work in the area of health. In the context of international psychology, we find the approach of Cuban health psychology particularly interesting as a possible model for discussions on health psychology in primary health care and psychological services in developing countries.

References

Garcia, L. (1980). Psychology and Health Care in Cuba. *American Psychologist,* **35**, 1090–1095.

Garcia-Averasturi, L. (1985). Community Health Psychology in Cuba. *Journal of Community Psychology,* **13**, 117–123.

Kristiansen, S. and Søderstrøm, K. (1987). *Cuban Health Psychology: A Description and Evaluation of the Role of Psychologists in the Cuban Health System, with Focus on the Activity in Primary Health Care* (Norwegian language). Thesis in Psychology, The Faculty of Psychology, University of Bergen.

Marin, B. V. (1985). Community Psychology in Cuba: A Literature Review. *Journal of Community Psychology,* **13**, s. 138–154.

MINSAP (1985). *Informe Anual.* Grupo Provincial de Psicologia, Ciudad de la Habana. Work-document.

MINSAP (1986). *Plan de Actividades de Psicologia para el Policlinico con el Medico de la Familia.* Havana: MINSAP.

Morales, F. (1984). La Psicologia: Insercion en Programas y Planes de Salud. Havana: Dirrecion Provincial de Salud. Work-document.

Morales, F. (1987). *Concideraciones Teoricas y Metodologicasacerca de la Especificidad de la Psicologia de la Salud.* Havana: Manuscript, unpublished.

Palacios, I. S. (1986). *Desempeno Profesional y Formacion del Psicologo en la Atencion Primaria.* Thesis in psychology. Havana: Instituto de Desarollo de la Salud, MINSAP.

SECTION TWO

TRAINING WITHIN HEALTH PSYCHOLOGY

CHAPTER 7

UNDERGRADUATE HEALTH PSYCHOLOGY: ANOTHER CHALLENGE FOR AN AMBITIOUS FIELD

THOMAS N. DORSEL

Francis Marion College

ANDREW BAUM

Uniformed Services University of the Health Sciences

Approaches to teaching undergraduate health psychology are explored drawing on information gathered from a national survey and from an APA symposium. Data from the survey are summarized, followed by brief descriptions of actual courses reflecting a range of approaches. Finally, a hypothetical course which blends the dominant features of existing courses is presented as a mainstream prescription for current development of undergraduate health psychology courses.

Health psychology has been a rapidly growing field. Hardly an issue of the *American Psychologist* or the *APA Monitor* appears without a significant contribution from the field of health psychology. Similarly, the Annual Convention of the American Psychological Association has regularly devoted major program tracks to health psychology, while journals and books have appeared and several professional societies now focus on some aspect of the association of behavior and health.

Not unexpectedly, the teaching of health psychology is commanding increased interest concurrent with advances being made in the research and clinical domains of the field. Considerable attention has already been given to doctoral and post-doctoral training as reflected in articles in *Health Psychology* (Belar, Wilson and Hughes, 1982; Belar and Siegel, 1983) and in the National Working Conference on Education and Training in Health Psychology (Matarazzo, 1983; Stone, 1983). More recently, attention has been directed toward instruction in health psychology at the undergraduate level as evidenced by a national survey conducted by the Council of Directors of Health Psychology Training and a symposium devoted to the topic at the 1986 Annual Convention of the American Psychological Association. The following is a summary of what was learned about current undergraduate activities in health psychology from the aforementioned survey and symposium.

RESULTS OF SURVEY CONDUCTED BY THE COUNCIL OF DIRECTORS OF HEALTH PSYCHOLOGY TRAINING

In 1986 the Council of Directors of Health Psychology Training undertook a survey to determine the extent of undergraduate instruction in health psychology and to compile a data base that might help programs develop such courses. A questionnaire asking for information about health psychology courses was developed, and approximately 1200 surveys were mailed to undergraduate programs in psychology. Of these, about half were returned; 109 schools reported that they had existing courses in health psychology; another 15 schools indicated that they offered a course covering health psychology topics, but that it was not solely concerned with the area; and 336 schools responded that they did not have a course at present, but many of these were in the process of developing one.

The survey asked respondents to provide a brief outline of the course or a listing of representative topics; the prerequisites, if any; whether the course was upper or lower division; how long it had been offered; how often it was offered; and the average enrollments. Respondents were also asked to list the texts and/or journal articles, films, and other resources used in the course, and were encouraged to send a syllabus.

Course level and prerequisites. Three-quarters of the courses were listed as "upper division" courses and most had prerequisites. Seventy-three percent required introductory or general psychology as a prerequisite, while only about 5% required social psychology, physiological psychology, statistics and methods, and/or abnormal psychology. Other prerequisites included introductory biology, developmental psychology, history and systems, personality, and behavioral analysis.

Course longevity and frequency. Courses in health psychology were, as one would expect, relatively new. About 27% of the courses had only been taught once, 12% twice, 26% three times, 10% four times, and 11% five times. The remaining 14% had been taught more often, ranging from six to fifteen times. Most courses (65%) were offered once each year, while approximately 15% were offered twice a year, with another 15% offered every other year.

Course organization and focus. Enrollments suggested seminars and small classes, as opposed to survey/lecture formats. Ten percent of the courses listed enrollments of 50 students or more, while the vast majority were in the 15–30 student range, and a substantial number listed enrollments of 6–15 students.

The basic orientation of the courses appeared to be along traditional lines regarding teaching methods, exams, and grading criteria. The syllabi tended not to emphasize topics of "personal relevance," but rather took a more "distant" approach suggesting that the courses were concerned with "psychological research dealing with health and illness," "applications of the theories and methods of psychology to health-related issues," and "application of psychological principles, methods, and processes to the assessment, prevention, maintenance and/or restoration of physical health."

Courses were organized around topical or problem areas rather than processes. Most emphasis seemed to be either on contributions of behavioral factors to illness, or on medically-relevant behavioral problems, such as compliance. Less attention was given to prevention and health promotion. To some extent this was due to the organization of the textbooks that were in use. Though they reflect a range of disciplinary perspectives, emphasis is on illness states or problems rather than on prevention and health.

Course titles. Of the courses reported, the majority (34%) were called "Health Psychology." Another 20% of the courses were titled "Behavioural Medicine" and the remaining course titles varied greatly. About 14% were either called "Stress" or "Stress Management," about 10% were called "Medical Psychology," and about 5% were titled "Social Psychology of Health." Other titles were used only once or twice and included "Psychology of Health and Illness," "Psychosocial Factors in Physical Illness," "Holistic Medicine," "Family Health Psychology," and "Community Health." Approximately 50 course titles were used. Though content of courses'varied somewhat, no consistent variation could be found for the primary course titles. That is, health psychology, behavioral medicine, and medical psychology courses tended to be very similar in content; and stress courses, despite their focus on stress and stress management, also included many of the same topics as did the other courses.

Course topics and textbooks. Course topics were varied and often listed under a number of names reflecting the same basic issues. Summarizing these topics and interpreting what a topic label meant in practice was not always easy. However, 50 syllabi provided outlines of course topics that could be analyzed to summarize the content of these courses. The remaining syllabi for courses in "health psychology," "medical psychology," or "behavioral medicine" provided textbook titles and/or guidelines for the course but did not include an outline of topics. The most frequently named topics were pain and pain management, compliance or adherence to medical regimen, and stress and illness, each included on more than half of the syllabi. Cardiovascular disease was covered in nearly half of the courses, and smoking, eating disorders/obesity, and illness behavior were included in just over 40% of the courses. A complete listing of course topics is presented in *Table 1.* Related to the issue of topics, the most commonly used textbooks at the time of the survey, along with the percentage of syllabi listing each of them, are presented in *Table 2*.

SPECIFIC EXAMPLES OF UNDERGRADUATE HEALTH PSYCHOLOGY COURSES

The following four course descriptions were presented at the 1986 Annual Convention of the American Psychological Association in a symposium entitled "The teaching of undergraduate health psychology." They represent a variety of orientations and approaches drawn from universities that vary in size and mission. In the following sections each course is briefly summarized, highlighting the differences among the offerings:

Broad-spectrum approach. Mary Ellen Olbrisch of the Medical College of Virginia described a senior seminar involving about 20 students. The purpose of the course was to provide an overview of the field of health psychology to include major

Table 1 Most frequently mentioned topics on submitted syllabi (the first ten were included on 50% or more of the syllabi, the next two on 25–49%, and the remaining topics on at least 10%). Approximately 50 other topics were mentioned, but at a rate of less than 10%

1. Pain and pain management	21. Learning theory
2. Stress and illness	22. Cognitive therapy
3. Compliance/Adherence with medical region	23. Alcohol use regimen
	24. Helplessness and Control
4. Cardiovascular disease	25. Models of illness
5. Smoking	26. Drug use/substance abuse
6. Eating	27. Nutrition
7. Illness behavior	28. Sleep/insomnia
8. Models of stress	29. Death and dying
9. Biofeedback	30. Placebo
10. Stress management	31. Headache
11. Type A behavior pattern	32. Patient-physician
12. Psychosomatic medicine	33. Surgery, psychological factors in surgery/medical exams
13. Psychoneuroimmunology	
14. History of behavioral medicine	34. Social support
15. Cancer	35. Coping with illness
16. Exercise	36. Assessment
17. Medical settings/hospitalization	37. Gastrointestinal disorders
18. Stress and coping	38. Practice of behavioral medicine
19. Behavioral factors in illness	39. Neuropsychology
20. Physiological bases of behavior	40. Prevention

research traditions and applications related to prevention and treatment. Teaching methods included readings, lectures, class discussions, laboratory activities, and guest speakers. Students were further encouraged to seek out professionals in the career areas to which they were aspiring in order to gain familiarity with important psychological issues regularly encountered in that setting.

Table 2 Percent of syllabi listing most commonly used texts

40% Gatchel R. J. and Baum A. (1983). *An Introduction to Health Psychology.* New York: Random House.

15% Cousins, N. (1979). *Anatomy of An Illness As Perceived By The Patient.* New York: W. W. Norton.

13% Taylor, S. E. (1985). *Health Psychology.* New York: Random House.

12% Greenberg, J. (1983). *Comprehensive Stress Management.*

9% APA. (1982). Behavioral Medicine. *Special Issue of Journal of Consulting and Clinical Psychology.*

7% Stone, G. C., Cohen, F. and Adler, N. E. (1979). *Health Psychology: A Handbook.* San Francisco: Josey-Bass.

7% Prokop, C. K. and Bradley, L. A. (Eds.) (1981). *Medical Psychology: Contributions to Behàvioral Medicine.* New York: Academic Press Academic Press.

7% Dimatteo, M. R. and Friedman, H. S. (1982). *Social Psychology and Medicine.* Cambridge: Oelgeschege, Gunn and Hain.

7% Davis, M., Eshelman, E. and McKay, M. *The Relaxation and Stress Reduction Workshop.* Richmond, CA: New Harbinger.

5% Gentry, W. D. (Ed.) *Handbook of Behavioral Medicine.*

5% Keefe, F. J. and Blumenthal, J. A. (1982). *Assessment Strategies in Behavioral Medicine.* New York: Grune and Stratton.

4% Pelletier, K. (1977). *Mind as Health/Mind as Slayer: A Holistic Approach to Preventing Stress Disorders.* New York: Elacorte/Lawrence.

4% Pelletier, K. (1979). *Holistic Medicine: From Stress to Optimum Health.* New York: New American Library.

4% Selye, H. (1978). *The Stress of Life.* New York: McGraw-Hill.

Behavioral medicine approach. Antonio E. Puente of the University of North Carolina at Wilmington described a junior-level course which concentrated on behavioral medicine. Students enrolled from the departments of psychology, nursing, biology and chemistry (mostly pre-medical students), sociology, medical technology, and business. Discussion of three basic topics served to introduce the course: (a) an analysis of behavioral principles and disease models, (b) psychological assessment of physical disorders, and (c) psychological change techniques applicable to behavioral medicine. The remainder of the course focused on a systematic analysis of major physical disorders. Guest speakers, films, and demonstrations were an integral part of the course, as well as a class project involving either a mini-internship, a self-oriented behavior-change project, survey research, and/or reviews of the literature.

Health promotion approach. William Bruce and Charles Prokop of the University of North Carolina at Asheville described a freshman, general-education course which focused on behavioral health. The purpose of the course was to provide a vehicle for the integration of health promotion with an undergraduate liberal arts education. The course included four topic areas related to prevention: (a) aerobic fitness, (b) stress and its management, (c) interpersonal relations and health, and (d) nutrition. Teaching methods included lectures, small group sessions, self-appraisal and self-contracting, as well as individual health promotion visits with a family-practice resident physician. Behavioral, physiological, and psychosocial measures were taken at the beginning and again at the end of the course resulting in several health-favorable changes for the health promotion students in comparison to controls.

Research approach. Richard Evans and his associates at the University of Houston described a junior-level course whose purpose was to introduce students to the general field of health psychology, and to give them an opportunity to work closely with a research team on a large-scale, field research project. The course was introduced with a two-week series of classes which, along with required and recommended readings, provided an overview of the field of health psychology. Students were then given an intensive four-week orientation to the research project. When the students actually began work on the research project, formal class meetings were held only occasionally, mainly to discuss developments within the research project itself. An optional guest lecture series involving current research areas in health psychology was also made available to the students during the course of the semester. Evaluation of student performance was based primarily on completion of the required research hours, and dependability regarding specific time and task commitments. Less critical, but considered for grading purposes, were attendance, participation, and periodic quizes covering reading and lecture materials.

A HYPOTHETICAL UNDERGRADUATE HEALTH PSYCHOLOGY COURSE BASED ON CURRENT PRECEDENTS

Considering the information presented above, a current, mainstream, undergraduate health psychology course would most likely be an upper division course with introductory psychology as a pre-requisite. It would range in enrollment from 15 to 30 students drawn from psychology and health-related majors, be taught once per year, and be titled "Health Psychology." The instructional methods used in the course would be fairly traditional, while common topics to be covered would include the following: Pain, stress, medical compliance, cardiovascular disease, smoking, eating, illness behavior, and biofeedback. The foci might range from being broad-spectrum, covering several areas of health psychology and applying these across a variety of career possibilities, to a more narrow concentration on more specific areas such as behavioral medicine, health promotion, or research approaches to the field. The course would likely draw on readings from a variety of sources.

CONCLUSION

Health psychology is a dynamic field reaching out for new frontiers. Current focus on undergraduate health psychology is yet another step in a natural progression regarding the dissemination of this new knowledge, a progression that is certain to proceed onto the secondary and elementary school levels, as well as to the public at large. As Michael Wertheimer, discussant in the aforementioned symposium noted, this is one of the best ways we can "give psychology away" (Miller, 1969).

Acknowledgments

Appreciation is extended to Ms. Kitti Virts for her assistance in the collection of the survey data and to Ms. Virginia Ridgill for assistance in the preparation of the manuscript.

References

Belar, C. D. and Siegel, L. J. (1983). A survey of post-doctoral training programs in health psychology. *Health Psychology*, **2,** 413–425.
Belar, C. D., Wilson, E. and Hughes, H. (1982). Health Psychology training in doctoral psychology programs. *Health Psychology*, **1,** 289–299.
Matarazzo, J. D. (1983). Education and training in health psychology: Boulder or bolder. *Health Psychology,* **2,** 73–113.
Miller, G.A. (1969). Psychology as a means of promoting human welfare. *American Psychologist*, **21,** 1063–1075.
Stone, G.C. (1983). National working conference on education and training in health psychology. *Health Psychology,* **2,** (no. 5, supplement), 1–153.

CHAPTER 8

ISSUES IN TRAINING CLINICAL HEALTH PSYCHOLOGISTS

CYNTHIA D. BELAR

Chief Psychologist and Clinical Director, Behavioral Medicine, Kaiser Permanente Medical Care Program, 4700 Sunset Boulevard, Los Angeles, USA

The author describes general issues in the training of clinical health psychologists and provides an overview of specific content needed in core health psychology and clinical health psychology assessment and intervention. Special attention is given to training in professional, personal, ethical and legal issues of practice.

Clinical health psychologists engage in the same broad range of functions as more traditional clinical psychologists, i.e., assessment, intervention, teaching, administration, consultation and research. The diversity of specific activities is immense. As examples, clinical health psychologists are known to:

a) assess candidates for suitability of penile prosthesis implants and cardiac transplant surgery;

b) provide treatment to enhance coping with pain, stressful medical/dental procedures, cancer and other illnesses;

c) design interventions to control symptoms such as vasospasms, incontinence, muscle spasms and vomiting;

d) provide behavior change programs for behavioral health risk factors such as smoking, weight and stress;

e) consult with hospital staff and administration to improve service delivery, enhance patient compliance and prevent staff burnout;

f) conduct research to assess cost-effectiveness of psychosocial treatment programs in health care settings and to identify high risk patients;

g) design psychosocial components of neurologic and cardiac rehabilitation programs;

h) train health care professionals in patient interviewing skills as well as psychosocial aspects of health and disease;

i) advocate for changes in governmental policies which impact health and disease.

Clinical health psychologists also use the range of diagnostic, therapeutic, consultation and research methods available to traditional clinical psychology. While they may reflect the variety of extant theoretical orientations, there is a basic commitment to a biopsychosocial model of health and disease. Obviously no one clinical health psychologist can be trained to become expert in all possible areas of practice. Thus in considering training issues, this paper will focus upon more generic issues of preparation for health psychology practice. An overview of the specific content required is provided, with some attention given to issues of professional conduct, ethics, malpractice and trainees' personal concerns. Each of these topics is more fully developed in the Belar, Deardorff and Kelly (1987) primer in clinical health psychology.

GENERAL TRAINING ISSUES

Fundamental to training in clinical health psychology is education in the broad discipline of psychology and training in basic clinical skills. The emphasis on core training in psychology and clinical practice stems from the fact that the field of health psychology is relatively new, and still dependent upon its underpinnings for basic nourishment and further growth. For example, the practitioner involved in direct services must have broad clinical assessment and treatment skills, including those in the area of psychopathology. While this author has heard it asserted that health psychologists deal with "normal" vs. "psychiatric" populations and thus do not need knowledge and skills in psychopathology, such is not the case. Medical–surgical populations have high base rates of problems such as anxiety and depression, and the general population itself has a significant base rate of psychopathology. The clinical health psychologist must be able to understand the *whole* patient in the context of his/her total biopsychosocial environment.

The practitioner needs training in research skills in order to critically evaluate research reports in this rapidly developing area, to conduct the program evaluations so often required for professional accountability, and to extend the knowledge base of clinical health psychology practice. Stan Maes' article in this volume more fully details issues concerning research training in health psychology.

In addition to core psychology training, the clinical health psychologist must obtain knowledge and skills in the following areas:†

a) social bases of health and disease
b) biological bases of health and disease
c) psychological bases of health and disease
d) health policy, systems and organizations
e) health assessment, consultation and intervention
f) health research methods
g) ethical, legal and professional issues associated with health psychology practice
h) interdisciplinary collaboration

Expertise can be developed through both coursework and field training experiences. However, to provide quality education and training in clinical health psychology the program must arrange for exposure to health care settings, a multidisciplinary faculty and experienced clinical health psychologists who can serve as mentors in the training process.

† These areas have been recommended by the National Working Conference on Education and Training in Health Psychology held in 1983 in New York, USA (Stone, 1983).

Courses specific to the health area which should be considered are those in anatomy and physiology, pathophysiology, applied pharmacology, health economics and health care systems. While the clinical health psychologist needs to understand disease, its treatment, course, prevention and outcome along with its psychosocial components, he/she must also understand the *context* within which the health care system operates. In some countries changes in health care delivery have been so dramatic that only the most recent references will suffice.

Courses in medical terminology are also useful. One must be able to understand the language of health care in order to communicate effectively. Trainee investment in a good medical dictionary and basic medical texts is worthwhile. In addition, the ability to decode medical abbreviations is a must if one wants to be able to read the medical chart of a referred patient. The goal of such education is *not* to become a "junior physician", but rather to be familiar enough with such material to be able to perform efficiently, communicate accurately, establish rapport, and inquire intelligently. It would also be wise to provide for training in cardiopulmonary resuscitation, as this is often required for work in health care settings. Suggested English language readings in clinical health psychology have been provided by Belar *et al.* (1987). Disease specific organizations (e.g., Arthritis Foundation) can provide a wealth of information on particular topics, and hospital libraries house audiovisual materials developed for continuing medical education.

However, didactic experiences are not sufficient training for clinical health psychology, as the wisdom acquired through clinical practice is not communicable in a purely didactic form. Indeed one of the hallmarks of professional training is the development of applied skills under the tutelage of "masters". Thus availability of appropriate role models, supervisors and mentors who are actively engaged in clinical health psychology is crucial to training.

Finally, exposure to health care systems facilitates comprehension of relevant sociopolitical features that can determine the difference between success and failure for the clinical health psychologist. Professional conduct is often as important as technical expertise in the delivery of effective professional services. Thus trainees need both role models and immersion in the health care system where they can also learn the unwritten rules of conduct.

ISSUES RELATED TO HEALTH CARE SETTINGS

Clinical health psychologists often practice in hospital, clinic or individual practice settings, thus training needs to insure sensitivity to the formal and informal aspects of these settings. For example, hospital practice is often regulated by very specific rules concerning personnel identification, medical record entries, professional practice privileges, and quality assurance. Governmental legislation often affects practice with respect to limits of patient confidentiality, professional licensure and reimbursement regulations. Understanding the informal aspects of health care settings such as referral customs and implicit power hierarchies also needs to be emphasized.

However, training programs need to avoid inappropriate "medical socialization" of psychologists. Elfant (1985) has described the tendency of physicians to attempt to "fix" people in a heroic, action-oriented, authoritarian, and rather imperialistic manner. The "good patient" is often the passive recipient of physician determined treatments. Elfant expressed concerns that health psychology practitioners will overidentify with this culture and forego the psychological treatment model that insists on the autonomy and freedom of choice of the patient. This concern is especially relevant to the use of behavioral interventions in order to enhance patient compliance to physician determined medical regimens. Health psychology training programs should explicitly address this aspect of trainee socialization, along with its implications for ethical practice.

PERSONAL ISSUES IN CLINICAL HEALTH PSYCHOLOGY TRAINING

In addition to specific content and professional behavior issues, training in clinical health psychology should also be sensitive to personal characteristics of trainees that may impact their professional behavior or their own satisfaction with clinical health psychology practice. Some individuals are not well-suited to the work, or have unrealistic expectations given some of the recent glamorization of the field. Mismatches are costly in terms of educational resources and emotional well-being, thus these issues should be examined early in the process of training.

Clinical health psychology trainees are likely to be confronted with death, disability and disfigurement that may trigger personal concerns or result in an inability to work effectively with certain populations (e.g., burn unit patients, head and neck surgery patients, cancer patients). Trainees may need encouragement to deal with personal issues related to body image and physical vulnerability; at a minimum a period of acclimation is needed (Belar, 1980). Desensitized faculty need to be sensitive to this issue without being overly intrusive into the personal life of the trainee.

Clinical health psychologists also have to learn to deal with the tensions found among the multiple health care disciplines. For example, although this varies across cultures, in the United States medicine continues to wield considerable power in health care. (Interestingly, with the growth of managed health care systems in the United States, business-related disciplines have become more prominent and present a new group of professionals with whom psychologists must learn to deal effectively.) Historically, psychologists have often felt treated as "second class citizens" as compared to physicians. Thus clinical health psychologists must have a high frustration tolerance and not be overly defensive in their professional relationships with physicians. As Shows (1976) has pointed out, readiness to project conflict into professional interactions can make collaborative efforts difficult. With time, experience, and savy mentors, trainees will learn about tensions among other disciplines and subspecialities (e.g., medicine and surgery), and learn effective methods of handling conflict in interdisciplinary relationships. However it is true that working in clinical health psychology often involves a forced dependency upon the expertise and performance of another profession, usually medicine or dentistry. Some individuals have special difficulties with this, especially when it involves dependence upon a profession of greater social status.

Finally, becoming aware of one's own stimulus value and its implications in patient contact and the health care setting is an especially important part of the supervisory process. A feature perhaps more unique in clinical health psychology than in traditional psychological practice is the visibility of maladaptive behavior (e.g., smoking, obesity). According to social learning theory, therapist modeling of good behavioral health is related to therapeutic effectiveness. Should a psychologist offer a smoking cessation program with a pack of cigarettes visible in his/her pocket, or be a smoker at all for that matter? Open discussion of professional conduct issues is an important part of the training program.

TRAINING IN HEALTH PSYCHOLOGY ASSESSMENT AND INTERVENTION

In assessing a problem, clinical health psychologists must understand interactions among the patient, the disease or medical procedure, and the person's environment. The biopsychosocial model is fundamental to the field, although theoretical orientations may vary. Training programs should provide skills in a broad range of assessment methods. Potential targets of assessment include the patient, the health care system, the family and the sociocultural context. The specific types of information obtained include biological/physical, affective, cognitive and behavioral. Methods of assessment include interview, questionnaires, diaries, psychometrics (both broad band and narrow-focus measures), observation, psychophysiological measurement and use of archival data. Fuller discussions of clinical health psychology assessment are found in Belar *et al.* (1987), Karoly (1985) and Keefe and Blumenthal (1982).

Some assessment methods, such as the Type A Structured Interview (Rosenman, 1978) and the Millon Behavioral Health Inventory (Millon, Green and Meagher, 1982) have been developed specifically for health psychology problems. In addition, depending upon the areas of practice in which skills are being trained, specific disease related measures might be incorporated into the curriculum (e.g., Arthritis Impact Measurement Scale [Meenan, Gertman & Mason, 1982]).

Other assessment methods, such as the Minnesota Multiphasic Personality Inventory (Hathaway and McKinley, 1967), were developed and normed on psychiatric populations and thus standard interpretations do not apply to medical–surgical populations. While many of the traditional psychological assessment tools can be useful in clinical health psychology practice, training should focus on the *appropriate* use of these techniques. Knowledge of relevant norms and interpretations based on clinical health psychology research is absolutely necessary in order to insure their appropriate use.

Training in health psychology interventions involves the selection of appropriate targets with respect to level of intervention (patient, family, health care system or sociocultural context) and domain of intervention (biological/physical, affective, cognitive, behavioral). The clinical health psychologist needs skills in utilizing a wide range of possible interventions including maximization of the placebo effect, supportive counseling, verbal psychotherapies, education and information, crisis intervention, relaxation training, imagery, hypnosis, biofeedback, systematic desensitization, modeling, skills training, contingency management, self-monitoring and cueing, and cognitive-behavioral therapies. For example, in order to provide comprehensive psychological care for a cancer patient, the psychologist might need to provide supportive counseling for the patient and his/her family, imagery training to increase quality of life; relaxation training to decrease the anticipatory nausea associated with chemotherapy, systematic desensitization for needle phobia, and existentially oriented psychotherapy for life review.

Training in clinical health psychology practice should also include a special focus on issues related to establishing rapport with medical–surgical patients who may, depending upon local culture, hold negative stereotypes related to obtaining psychological services, and who may be less than appreciative of their physician's referral to one.

ISSUES RELATED TO ETHICAL BEHAVIOR AND PROFESSIONAL MALPRACTICE

Professional training also requires attention to ethical issues in practice. Clinical health psychology involves unique ethical issues due to the special settings and patient populations encountered. For example, there is increased responsibility for physical health given the nature of populations served; concomitant medical evaluations and management must be assured. Yet because psychologists usually work alongside other health professionals delivering care, there is also increased risk for diffusion of responsibility for health care. Boundaries of professional competence, the need to maintain current knowledge, and an obligation to obtain relevant consultation/supervision are all ethical issues requiring attention.

Likewise, the psychologist must often take special measures to protect patient confidentiality in the hospital setting, given the lack of privacy in hospital rooms and the availability of medical charts to hospital staff. The patient must be informed about the *limits* of confidentiality for practice to be ethical. Informed consent also requires that psychologists convey information about possible conflicts of interest to the patient. Not infrequently services are requested by a third party whose priority might be quite different from that of the patient (e.g., family members' request to insure patient compliance to a medical regimen, physician's desire to obtain a release for an organ transplant).

Another issue previously discussed is the need to recognize personal problems which may interfere with professional effectiveness. Actual harm could be done by a psychologist who unwittingly expressed revulsion at the sight of a postmastectomy patient. Finally, an important ethical issue has to do with appropriate public statements regarding findings in the area of clinical health psychology. Exaggerated claims of treatment effectiveness and overstated relationships among psychological variables and health outcomes will lead not only to a public backlash when the field cannot deliver, but guilt and negative reactions among patients who "fail" to exert psychological control over their diseases. Training in the appropriate presentation of the field to the public and to consumers is essential.

Malpractice risks in clinical health psychology also need attention during training. A significant malpractice risk is the inadvertent practice of medicine without a license. While laws regarding this will vary, it is unlikely that recommendations regarding use of medication and diagnoses of physical health problems will be viewed as within the scope of licensed practice for psychologists. Thus the wording of recommendations to patients and clinical diagnoses in reports must not reflect such practices. For example, the psychologist should not advise a patient to decrease antihypertensive medication, or diagnose migraine headache. Appropriate medical consultation must be obtained and documented in the clinical record.

Knapp and VandeCreek (1981) suggest that the clinical health psychologist has more malpractice risks than the traditional mental health service provider. They assert that medical surgical patients are more likely to claim that physical harm (vs. emotional harm) has been the result of the health psychology practice. In the courts, physical health damage is viewed as easier to prove than emotional damage.

Secondly, because many cases do not provide for continuing contact over time with the patient, the clinical health psychologist often does not have the close emotional bond with patients that the traditional psychotherapist has the opportunity to develop. Many patients experience only brief contacts with the health psychologist. Knapp and VandeCreek believe that a close therapist–patient relationship serves to deter malpractice suits in traditional areas of practice.

In the author's experience, perhaps the most frequent grounds ffor legitimate malpractice suits in clinical health psychology involve the misuse of psychometric instruments. This can occur through the use of inappropriate norms/interpretations for particular measures, or through the use of psychometric techniques to conclude that physical symptoms are "functional" in nature.

In summary, the field of clinical health psychology and its perspectives on training are still evolving. The heterogeneity that exists reflects the broadness of the field. However, core education and training for all clinical health psychologists includes fundamental courses in the discipline of psychology and the study of relationships/applications of these fundamentals to health, disease, the health care delivery system, and health policy-making. Clinical health psychology training also includes specific methods of health assessment and intervention, with special attention paid to professional issues, ethical principles and legal aspects of practice. Necessary components of programs include a multidisciplinary faculty, relevant applied settings and accomplished mentors/supervisors.

References

Belar, C. D. (1980). Training the clinical psychology student in behavioral medicine. *Professional Psychology*. **11**, 596–604.

Belar, C. D., Deardorff, W. W. and Kelly, K. E. (1987). *The practice of clinical health psychology*. New York: Pergamon Press.

Elfant, A. B. (1985). Psychotherapy and assessment in hospital settings: Ideological and professional conflicts. *Professional Psychology: Research and practice*. **16**, 55–63.

Hathaway, S. R. and McKinley, J. C. (1967). *The Minnesota Multiphasic Personality Inventory Manual*. New York: Psychological Corporation.

Karoly, P. (Ed.) (1985). *Measurement strategies in health psychology*. New York: John Wiley & Sons.

Keefe, F. J. and Blumenthal, J. A. (Eds.) (1982). *Assessment strategies in behavioral medicine*. New York: Grune & Stratton.

Knapp, S. and VandeCreek, L. (1981). Behavioral medicine: Its malpractice risks for psychologists. *Professional Psychology*, **12**, 677–683.

Meenan, R. F., Gertman, P. M. and Mason, J. H. (1982). The arthritis impact measurement scales: Further investigation of a health status measure. *Arthritis and Rheumatology*. **25**, 1048–1053.

Millon, T., Green, C. J. and Meagher, R. B. (1982). *Millon Behavioral Health Inventory Manual*. Minneapolis: National Computer Systems.

Rosenman, R. (1978). The interview method of assessment of the coronary-prone behavior pattern. In T. M. Dembroski, S. M. Weiss, J. L. Shields, S. G. Haynes and M. Feinleib (Eds.), *Coronary-prone behavior*. New York: Springer-Verlag.

Shows, W. D. (1976). Problem of training psychology interns in medical schools: A case of trying to change the leopard's spots. *Professional Psychology*. **7**, 393–395.

Stone, G. C. (Ed.) (1983). National working conference on education and training in health psychology. *Health Psychology*, **2** (Suppl. 5), 1–153.

CHAPTER 9

TRAINING RESEARCH HEALTH PSYCHOLOGISTS

S. MAES and F. KITTEL

Clinical and Health Psychology Section, Leiden University, P.O. Box 9555 2300 RB Leiden, The Netherlands

This article comprises two parts.

In the first part, some general issues related to research training are discussed, including the "Scientist–Practitioner Model," training for basic and applied research, differences between the USA and Europe at various levels of training, and types or areas of research students should be trained for.

In the second part, seven specific objectives of research training are discussed. These objective are (a) learning to write a review of the research literature, (b) learning to critically evaluate a journal article, (c) learning to plan and carry out a specific health psychology research study, (d) learning to communicate, (e) learning to enhance co-operation of professionals in the field, (f) learning to raise funds, (g) learning to respect ethical issues.

1. SOME GENERAL ISSUES

1.1 *The Scientist–Practitioner Model*

Above all we are of the opinion that research health psychologists should never be trained in research alone, as well as health psychologists working in practical settings should always receive basic research training.

This point of view is, however, far from being new, as it was first expressed in 1949 at the Boulder Conference, which introduced the concept of the scientist–practitioner, implying that those who are trained to provide service must be adequately trained in conducting research (Matarazzo, 1983; Singer, 1987). Conversely, apart from core psychology training, health psychology researchers should acquire practical skills. The reason for this is that health psychology research does not take place in a vacuum but, more often than not, in an ecologically valid or service delivery setting. Among these skills the following may be mentioned: assessment, intervention, consultation and training skills. For a discussion of training issues related to these skills we refer the reader to the article by Cynthia Belar in this volume.

1.2 *Basic and Applied Research*

There is no good reason why training for basic and applied research in health psychology should be distinguished. Firstly, the distinction is, more often than not, based on arbitrary criteria, such as: (a) basic research is conducted in the laboratory, applied research in real life settings; (b) basic research contributes more to the theoretical-concept than to the applied domain, and (c) applied studies are less well controlled, despite the potentially greater applicability of the results (Singer, 1987). As one can think of well controlled studies that take place in ecologically valid settings and contribute to both the theoretical and practical aspects of a discipline, the distinction is rather academic.

What is more important for training purposes, is that the techniques of conducting research studies do not substantially differ between so-called basic and applied research. In other words, whether a research study is a basic or an applied one, has much more to do with the attributions made by the outside world than with objective criteria. From this point of view, applied research could be defined as research which is either of direct interest to or initiated by a specific group in society, other than the investigator (Singer, 1987). In other words we fully agree with Miller (1987, p. 75) that ". . . in health psychology the requirements for training in basic or applied research in the laboratory or in the field have many more similarities than differences." As a consequence, we are of the opinion that there should be no differentiation in training for basic and applied research.

1.3 *American Structuralism Versus European Craftsmanship*

From an American perspective, there should be no systematic training in health psychology at the undergraduate level (Stone, 1983). Although still very few European training programmes in health psychology exist (Tilburg, Leiden and Utrecht in the Netherlands, Surrey and London in the U.K., and a national programme in the Flemish part of Belgium are at present the only established), these programmes are in contrast to the American scene, as they are offered at master's level and can be completed in two years. It should be noted, however, that each of these programmes includes a research based thesis.

The differences between the American and European models of training become even more apparent at the doctoral level. Generally speaking, with the exception of the United Kingdom, where formal programmes do exist, there are no formal training programmes in psychology at the doctoral level in most European countries. Postgraduate education for research psychologists takes place in virtually every European university where graduate programmes in psychology exist. However, most of these programmes follow an apprenticeship model, implying that students must produce a research based doctoral dissertation under the supervision of a university professor. The apprenticeship may extend over a long period of time. The American model, on the other hand, is very formal: a doctoral degree is obtained after completion of a four to five year study programme, which includes a dissertation.

In Europe, the doctoral level is considered the final degree of training. In contrast, however, many in the United States are of the opinion that "the degree of sophistication needed to conduct independent research in health psychology can rarely be achieved in a doctoral programme alone" (Friedman, 1987, p. 361). According to the American Working Conference on Health Psychology Training (Stone, 1983, pp. 137–138), "three basic mechanisms of training apply at the post-doctoral level: (a) formal courses and/or seminars, the extent of which depends upon the extent of predoctoral training in health psychology: (b) the apprenticeship model that involves a one-to-one relationship with a mentor as a postdoctoral student conceptualizes and implements a line of research and (c) participation in an ongoing research programme that the postdoctoral student has not had a role in conceptualizing will allow development of area skills relevant to health psychology, as he or she joins in an existing research team." As there seems to be a heterogeneity across and within these programmes, there is no prototypical programme which can be described here (Belar, 1987).

In conclusion, the American and European models of training differ greatly. Where some may think this is a question of development, in our opinion, it is rather the consequence of two different worlds or philosophies. At the base of the American model is the idea that organized and formal forms of learning are the best guarantee for producing highly qualified researchers (Maher, 1983). Behind the European model is a long tradition, which may originate from medieval times when a craftsman could only become a master after a long period of apprenticeship and at the approval of the existing Masters of the Guild to which he belonged. In this model, the quality of the product ("mastery") is the principal criterion for obtaining any postgraduate degree.

Both these models may have advantages as well as disadvantages. The main disadvantage of the European model is that only the happy few acquire a doctorate, as it requires, for motivational and other reasons, devoting many years to producing a "masterpiece" for acceptance by a scientific establishment. In other words, the European model certainly fails to produce numbers. In addition, since there are no European standards for research training at doctoral level, quality control is difficult. On the other hand, the American model guarantees that larger numbers of students starting predoctoral education will acquire a Ph.D. In terms of efficiency, the American model is, without any doubt, superior. As for quality, the main advantage and disadvantage of any formal educational system is that most students are encouraged to finish their degree, which they usually do with varying success. In other words, numbers may also be dangerous (Maher, 1983).

In general, any form of training for research health psychologists at the doctoral level should include at least a four year apprenticeship period under the tutelage of an experienced senior scientist. This apprenticeship should lead to one or a series of publications which meet international scientific standards. This advanced level of training is the minimum level required to start independent research or to function as an independent researcher in a multidisciplinary team. European universities should at least consider including obligatory courses in advanced research design, methodology, statistics and computer skills at the doctoral level. Where such courses are lacking, senior staff members should encourage forms of peer teaching. On completion of the advanced level, fellows should be encouraged to spend at least one year with a research group in another country or state. This may apply more to the European than to the American scene, as it is seen as a form to complement possible training biases at a doctoral level in a situation where international training standards are lacking. At the same time, such stays may also help to minimize the "language" and "cultural" barriers in Europe, which can sometimes jeopardize collaboration on a European level. The EEC's recent Erasmus programme is a very good initiative in this direction, as the aim of Erasmus (European Community Action Scheme for the Mobility of University Students) is to favor student and/or staff mobility between universities in the different member states.

1.4 *For what Type of Research should Students be Trained?*

Another fundamental question concerns the type of research students should become familiar with. The answer to such a question can be given by both a theoretical and practical point of view.

A theoretical point of view is represented by the classification of psychological studies by Stone (1979), shown in *Table 1*. In a recent publication, Stone (1987) documents that the existing health psychology research focusses mainly on studies regarding the health target and health care processes, while largely neglecting all other research areas related to organizational or system issues. In addition, after examining manuscripts submitted to the journal "Health Psychology," the same author (Stone, 1987) found that less than 20% of these involved physiological measures as either independent or dependent variables.

In a survey conducted by the first author of this article (Maes, 1988) in 1987 on European research in life-styles and health, 216 health psychology research projects, spread over ten different Western-European countries were identified. A closer look

Table 1 Classification of Psychological Studies of the Health System (Stone, 1979).

I. *Studies of the health target*
- A. Psychobiological
  1. Effects of behaviour on body processes
  2. Effects of body abnormalities on behaviour
- B. Health behaviour
  1. Self-destructive behaviour
     drug abuse; accident proneness
  2. Preventive health behaviour
  3. Illness behaviour
     utilization; delay in treatment
  4. Sick role behaviour
     adherence; coping with stress of treatment
  5. Adjustment to chronic illness

II. *Studies of the health care system*
- A. Health care processes
  1. Outreach
  2. Diagnosis
  3. Prescribing; preparing patients for surgery
  4. Provider-patient interactions
- B. Treatment settings and devices
  1. Health care organizations
  2. Human factors
  3. Psychoarchitectural studies
- C. Health care careers
  1. Recruitment; specialty selection
  2. Training
  3. Stresses of health careers

III. *Planning and resources mobilization*

IV. *Studies of hazard reduction*

From: Stone, G. C. (1979). Psychology and the health system. In Stone, G. C., Cohen, F. and Adler, N. *Health psychology: A Handbook.* San Francisco: Jossey Bass.

Reprinted by permission

at these projects revealed that about half were related to psychological aspects such as stress, type-A behaviour, and psychosomatic topics. In contrast, however, with the exception of smoking, less than one third were related to research concerning habits such as: nutrition, weight, physical exercise, alcohol abuse, drug abuse, dental hygiene, sexual and driving behaviour, which have proven to be more closely related to morbidity and mortality. Furthermore, almost 80% were unifactorial (= related to one life-style aspect only). The rest were multifactorial. Of these multifactorial studies, about 60% were related to primary prevention. In addition, less than 10% of the total number of studies seemed to be prospective studies, the others being cross-sectional or intervention studies.

In brief, there are enormous biases in the existing research, some of which may endanger the future (funding) of health psychology research. The general impression is that health psychology research is too psychological or, in other words, neglects the fact that health psychology research is only part of a large interdisciplinary field of health and health care research. As such, future research should, among other things, take the above mentioned into account.

Apart from this more theoretical approach, one must not forget that any training programme is a preparation for jobs in the community. An informal survey carried out by the first author among Dutch health psychologists revealed that most of their jobs implied (at least partly) research skills, but that these skills can differ substantially, depending on their employment, which ranged, for example, from psychology departments to medical departments, interdisciplinary research institutes, patient organizations, community health care centres, rehabilitation centres, general hospitals, schools for health personnel and national health bodies. In other words, training programmes should be constructed based on data about what skills are actually needed. Many university training programmes suffer from the effects of Murphy's Law ("never ask a university teacher how much he or she would like to teach"). From this point of view, it is our impression that many training programmes may be easily overloaded with irrelevant content, resulting in the demotivation of students. Consequently, the content of research orientated courses and practica, at both the basic and advanced training level in health psychology, should not exclusively be determined by standard research textbooks, or theoretical frameworks, but also by what research health psychologists really do or could do. A survey to determine the most common topics, designs, methodology and statistics used in health psychology research could be a more solid basis for motivating students to do research than many of the present courses, which are not always ecologically valid. In addition, it should be a must that these courses be given by experienced research health psychologists, who are familiar with the field, rather than by methodologists.

2. SPECIFIC TRAINING OBJECTIVES

In this part of the article, we will identify and discuss seven objectives which should be met differentially at the various levels of research training.

2.1 *Learning to Write a Review of the Research Literature.*

One of the most obvious requirements is that students must be able to write a review of the existing research related to a specific health psychology topic. This implies being able to: (a) define the topic; (b) carry out a search in the Psychological Abstracts and/or Excerpta Medica files; (c) formulate criteria to decide which material to include and which not to include; (d) give a fair description of each relevant study, including research questions, population, methods, results and comments; (e) present the different studies in a (chrono)logical order; (f) make use of overview tables representing key features of the studies included and (g) write a conclusion and discussion in which general trends are summarized, explanations are offered for controversial findings, and guidelines for future research are formulated.

As far as the results are concerned, an alternative for the traditional review is the more quantitative meta-analysis, which allows one to condense the results of independent studies into a simple statistic—the average effect size for all major dependent variables. The effect size is the difference between the means of the experimental and the control groups divided by the standard deviation of the control group.

In order to reach this objective: (a) literature related to the existing health psychology courses should contain good examples of both review types; (b) practical classes should be organized in which these examples are discussed with the help of a comprehensive check-list (see, for example, Holt, 1977; Polgar and Thomas, 1988) and (c) during the programme, students should write at least two traditional review papers under the supervision of a senior health psychology staff member. In addition, as meta-analysis is becoming increasingly popular, they should at least once co-operate in small groups in order to carry out a meta-analysis on a specific health psychology topic.

2.2 *Learning to Critically Evaluate a Specific Journal Article*

A minimal objective in terms of research skills is that every student should be able to critically evaluate a specific journal article. However, training programmes do not always devote enough time to this topic.

As it is impossible here to include all the characteristics of a research study to be checked when evaluating a journal article, we wish to refer the reader to existing checklists which can be used for this purpose (Allen, 1973; Holt, 1977; Maher, 1978; Kratwohl, 1985; Polgar and Thomas, 1988). It should be noted that these checklists can also be used for preparing a research proposal. According to Kratwohl (1985), one could make a distinction between the evaluation of constraints (e.g. resource limits, institutional constraints or ethical aspects), which are neglected in the report of a study too often, and criteria to optimize the study (e.g. aspects of question choice and formulation, weighing of internal and external validity, credibility with the audience, information yield and resource allocation). Internal validity implies: credibility of explanation offered for central research questions, adequate translation of these explanations in operational questions or hypotheses, adequate demonstration of relationships found, elimination of rivalling explanations for the research findings, and credibility of the results. External validity implies: generality of the offered explanation, translation generality, demonstrated generality, elimination of restrictive explanations and replicability of the results.

It is obvious that, in order to achieve this objective, practical classes under the supervision of an experienced health psychology researcher should be organized. In addition, using an extensive checklist to help them, students should go through the process of preparing a research proposal.

2.3 *Learning to Plan and Carry Out a Specific Health Psychology Research Study*

One of the main requirements of virtually all health psychology programmes, including European master's programmes, is that students must be able to carry out a research study under the supervision of a senior staff member. For the European master's level, six months to a year seems to be the time limit, while the preparation of a doctorate dissertation may imply one to several years in the USA, and five year or more in Europe. As a consequence, it is impossible to formulate mutual criteria. However, programme includes mastering the following skills up to a certain level: (a) adequately describing the purpose of the study, including its theoretical, social and/or practical relevance; (b) summarizing the relevant research literature, including significant differences between the studies included; (c) formulating specific research questions and/or hypotheses based on previous studies or theory; (d) adequately selecting the design of the study (survey, experimental, quasi-experimental, epidemiological); (e) selecting and/or constructing measures; (f) defining and/or constructing a treatment, if appropriate; (g) collecting data, including adequate recruitment and assignment of subjects; (h) delivering, ensuring or controlling the delivery of a treatment, if appropriate; (i) analyzing the data in an appropriate way; (j) reporting the study in an adequate way, including a description of the purpose and relevance of the study, a summary of the relevant research literature, description of research questions, population, method, results and discussion (including interpretation and generalization of the results); and (k) critically evaluating one's own study, pointing out the weaknesses that should be overcome in future research.

In order to reach this objective, supervision is necessary at all levels. At master's level, close supervision of a small study is required. As a consequence, students at Tilburg University are, for example, not at liberty to choose their own research topics. Their project must be part of the research being carried out at the Health Psychology Section, since this seems the only way to respect time constraints and guarantee the quality of the supervision, which is crucial at this stage. Leaving students on their own at an early stage of the learning process not only affects the quality of the product, but also the student's motivation to engage in research positions. This scene was typical, at least in continental Europe, for many clinical psychologists who, as a consequence, lost the esteem of their academic colleagues and also failed to document the effectiveness of their interventions endangering their own jobs. Health psychologists should not make the same mistake.

As health psychology is at the intersection of many domains and disciplines beyond the knowledge and skills peculiar to psychology, the research health psychologist at doctoral level should also become familiar with several other health related specialties. This implies knowledge and skills in bio-statistics, computer science, epidemiology and public health. The trainee should not only be familiar with the traditional parametric and non-parametric univariate analyses, but also with the appropriate multivariate analyses (e.g. discriminant, multiple regression, factor, cluster and lisrel analyses, analyses of variance and covariance, log linear and multiple logistic, survival and life table analyses, and the Cox Model of Proportional Hazards).

Furthermore, besides the basic knowledge of file handling and data processing, the trainee should be able to manage statistical packages such as SPSS or BMDP or SAS, which are the most common.

In addition, the health psychology researcher should be thoroughly impregnated with epidemiological terminology, definitions and concepts, and be able to make a clear distinction between and within the following categories linked with: (a) description of targets/populations: impairment, disability, handicap, sickness, disease, illness—exposed vs nonexposed; (b) properties of data: indicators, determinants, markers, factors, variables; (c) characteristics of measurements and investigations: sensitivity, specificity, validity, repeatability, feasibility; (d) type of studies: descriptive, analytical or intervention epidemiological studies (primary, secondary, tertiary prevention); (e) calculations performed on data: proportions, rates, ratios—relative, attributable, multiple risks; (f) limitations of studies: nonrespondents, drop outs, raw data (not adjusted or standardized), various biases, effects (healthy worker, halo, placebo); (g) interpretation of findings: direct, indirect, causal association.

Next, in order to perform realistic relevant research, they must know: (a) where to find the information: libraries—World Health Organization (WHO), International Labour Organization (ILO), National Institutes of Health (NIH), European Economic Community (EEC); (b) how to obtain the information from medical or psychological indexes and excerpts or by an on-line retrieval (MEDLARS, MEDLINE); (c) the existence of research centres, specific to their topic and general establishments at both international and regional level delivering vital statistics; (d) the potential funding establishments. Consequently, they should be able to choose an adequate design: (a) survey: cross-sectional (prevalence), case-control (retrospective), cohort (prospective); (b) experimental: natural; quasi-experimental, controlled or randomised controlled carried out in single, double, triple blind, factorial or matching. In a next step, they should be able to choose the appropriate sample: cluster, grab, probability simple—random or stratified random, systematic, haphazard, or by quota. Finally, trainees should be capable of making an evaluation of their own study in terms of structure, process and out-comes by cost benefit, cost utility or cost effectiveness analyses.

It is obvious that the mastery of so many skills requires a long period of training, irrespective of the model of training (apprenticeship, formal courses or participation) used. It is, however, our conviction that learning by doing is important to become a good researcher. Skills should, whenever possible, not be taught independently, but related to the specific research study being carried out by (or in co-operation with) the student. Formal programmes especially run the risk of violating this basic philosophy, as teaching may then become a more important objective than students' learning. In addition, at an advanced level, close contact with other researchers in the same area is necessary for further development. Too many researchers think at a specific moment in time that "they know how to do it, and even better than most of their colleagues". This individualism of researchers, a consequence of which can sometimes be that even researchers within the same group or department are either uninformed or ill-informed about each other's research, is, in our opinion, the cause of the fact that many experienced researchers know more and more about less and less. As a consequence the next objective is vital.

2.4 *Learning to Communicate*

Students should be fully trained in several means of communication. First of all, adequate communication requires knowledge related to health and disease and the health care system. As a consequence, essential medical knowledge with respect to processes, assessment and treatment of various health problems, and knowledge concerning the organizations of the health care system must be gained by future researchers, as without this knowledge, successful communication with other academics is not possible. In addition, every form of research also implies getting in touch with many and various other individuals, groups or establishments such as government or regional organizations, leading staff in enterprises, schools, army, hospitals, labour unions, occupational physicians etc. It, therefore, seems relevant to train the student in methods of negotiation.

Preparing a written report of a study is mentioned earlier in this paper as an important objective. It would be wise to add hereto training in oral communication skills—another way of exchanging experience and findings. Particular emphasis should be placed on the ability to speak in public and to deliver clear visual messages (slides, overheads).

Conferences, congresses, workshops etc. are places where formal presentations are delivered. Here the future research worker has, through informal communication, the opportunity to speak with other researchers of the same domain, and thus the possibility to foster international co-operation.

2.5 *Learning to Enhance Co-Operation of Professionals in the Field*

As Singer (1987) pointed out, training researchers in practical skills increases the credibility of the researcher among his professional colleagues. It has also been demonstrated that, these practical skills can even be used to offer compensation to the practical setting where research is, more often than not, experienced as an additional burden (Maes and Grauenkamp, 1982). For example, when a researcher can function as part of a team or offer co-operating help with practical tasks, professional colleagues will accept the extra workload which goes with the implementation and the carrying out of a research project more readily. As such, the more skills a researcher acquires, the greater his/her credibility, and the stronger his/her negotiating position. Other advantages of these skills are mentioned in the article by Cynthia Belar (this issue) when she discusses personal issues in clinical health psychology training. Another important aspect is that there should be continuous communication between the researcher and health care personnel in the field from a very early to the final stage of the research process. This not only increases the commitment of practitioners to research projects, but also guarantees the social reference and the feasibility of the study and applicability of the findings.

2.6 *Learning to Raise Funds*

This objective deserves more attention than it probably receives in many training programmes. This is best demonstrated by the results of a survey on research activities in psychology, which was mailed some years ago to a stratified random sample of 9,991 American resident APA members. A total of 6,551 usable surveys were returned. Approximately half the sample proved to be involved in research activities. Of these, only 42% were involved in funded research activities. When researchers without funding were asked why they did not have funding, the most important reasons were: because their research was not on a large enough scale to require funding; because they did not have enough time to prepare proposals, and because they believed that the chances of a proposal being accepted were slight.

In addition, when funded and non-funded researchers were asked about the sources of information on research funding, the two groups appeared to differ substantially in the amount of sources used. This is best illustrated by the fact that 43.8% of the funded researchers used personal contracts with funding agency personnel, while only 16.1% of the non-funded researchers used such personal contacts. In addition, those who reported funded research published much more than those not reporting funded research (Lowman and Stapp, 1981).

Although this survey was conducted in the USA, and concerns psychological research in general, it is our conviction that the results are, mostly likely, also valid for the European scene, and also apply to health psychology research. As a consequence, students should be taught to write research proposals, if possible on the official forms used by various research funding bodies. The already mentioned checklists may be of great help to both the graduate and the advanced student. In addition, students should be asked to construct lists with relevant funding agencies in the area of health psychology. This way they become familiar with the existent (or non-existent) information on funding. At an advanced level they should assist a senior health psychology researcher through the whole process of raising funds for a specific research project. Too many researchers consider their expertise in fund raising the legitimate secret of a good cook. These so-called secrets may imply active inquiries at various funding bodies, including personal contacts with the personnel of these agencies. As such, junior researchers may discover that many of these people actively assist a researcher in the process of fund raising, and that the chances of obtaining funds are only with those who apply for them.

2.7 *Learning to Respect Ethical Issues*

In her book on understanding psychological research, Miriam Lewin (1979) tackles ethical issues. She mentions that research should rest upon considered judgment about how best to contribute to psychological science and human welfare.

Her "ten commandments" for ethical psychological research also apply to health psychology research and can be summarized as follows: (a) the investigators are personally responsible for making a careful evaluation of the ethical acceptability of their study, and weighing scientific and human values in terms of costs and benefits; (b) the investigators are also responsible for the ethical treatment of research participants by collaborators, assistants, students and employees all of whom however incur parallel obligations; (c) the investigators have to inform the participant of all features of the research that might be expected to influence willingness to participate, and explain all other aspects of the research about which the participant inquires. This in order to obtain an *informed consent*; (d) *openness and honesty* are essential characteristics when the methodological requirements of a study necessitate concealment or deception, the investigators are required to ensure the participants' understanding of the reasons for this action; (e) the investigators have to respect the *individual's freedom* to decline or discontinue; (f) a clear and fair agreement between the investigators and the research participants must be made. The investigators are obliged to honour all processes and commitments included in that agreement. Research subjects have ethical obligations too, namely to keep appointments and to be frank with the researcher. This principle deals with *fairness and freedom from exploitation*; (g) the investigators have to *protect* participants from *physical and mental discomfort, harm and danger*. If the risk of such consequences exists, the investigators are required to inform the participant; (h) after the data are collected, the investigators have to provide the participant with a full description of the nature of the study and to remove any misconceptions that may have arisen, what could be called *debriefing;* (i) when research procedures may result in undesirable consequences for the participant, the investigators are responsible for detecting and *removing or correcting* these *negative consequences*, those being either short or long-term; (j) the anonymity of research should be strictly maintained. Information is *confidential*.

From a practical point of view, however, the following comments must be made concerning the ethical issue:

a) As already mentioned, when studying human beings, one must obtain consent from the subjects selected, and guarantee anonymity and confidentiality. This, however, will not facilitate the work of the health psychologist in terms of linking data of surveys made at different intervals. This is particularly true in countries where medical ethics are very strict, the consequence is, for example, that it is difficult to set up registers to record morbidity incidence.

b) In an experimental design, the intervention is an action imposed on the subjects by the researcher, whereas the absence of intervention (e.g. in the control group) is an action imposed by "nature"—usually deleterious for the less "favoured" groups or individuals. If we look at the present state of knowledge, the following questions arise: "On the one hand are we researchers allowed to intervene without being really aware of all possible counter-effects? On the other hand, if we think that an intervention has a positive effect on people's health and no harmful effect, are we allowed to perform an actual controlled trial?" The United States were confronted earlier with this problem and it explains the emergence of usual care groups (instead of no-care groups) for the comparison with specific care groups (Multiple Risk Factor Intervention Trial Research Group, 1982).

c) A final issue in terms of ethics is related to the researchers' own results and findings. In addition to presenting possible results, whether they be positive, invalid or negative, the researcher must keep the appropriate claims as to these results in mind: exaggerated optimism or pessimism can have deleterious effects.

From a training point of view, in our experience these different aspects are best taught by asking students to think of as many violations of ethical issues as possible related to their own research study. In order to discover how many of these violations can be made by a naive researcher, a few tutorial group sessions, supervised by a senior researcher, should be devoted to the exchange of "interesting violations". In addition, students should be taught to bring violations out into the open, including them in their publications whenever they are discovered in their own research.

References

Allen, G. R. (1973). The graduate student's guide to theses and dissertation: A practical manual for writing and research. San Francisco: Jossey-Bass.

Belar, C. D. (1987). The current status of predoctoral and postdoctoral training in health psychology. In G. C. Stone *et al.* (Eds.) *Health Psychology: A Discipline and a Profession* (pp. 325–334). Chicago: The University of Chicago Press.

Friedman, H. S. (1987). Postdoctoral training for research. In G. C. Stone *et al.* (Eds.) *Health Psychology: A Discipline and a Profession* (pp. 361–369). Chicago: The University of Chicago Press.

CHAPTER 10

TRAINING IN HEALTH PSYCHOLOGY: AN INTERNATIONAL LOOK

GERDA J. METHORST, MARY A. JANSEN
and AD J. F. M. KERKHOF

*Department of Clinical, Health and Personality Psychology,
University of Leiden, Leiden, The Netherlands*

With the progression of health psychology as a new field in psychology specific training programs are more and more needed. A survey of the training situation of health psychology in Northern America, Europe, Australia, and New Zealand highlighted a lack of formalized training programs in most countries except the United States and Canada, as well as an enormous variety between countries on standards of training, and on the differentiation of health psychologists from clinical psychologists.

For the qualification of health psychology as an independent psychological discipline a plea is made for international standardization of quality control and suggestions for the content of formalized training programs in health psychology are given.

INTRODUCTION

The field of health psychology has progressed rapidly since its inception in the late 1970's. This development has been chronicled by Stone (this issue) and as he notes, until now health psychologists have come primarily from two sources: psychologists originally trained as researchers with interests related to health, and psychologists originally trained as clinicians with interests in applying their clinical expertise to problems in health care. Because the field is relatively new it is only recently that questions have been raised about how health psychologists should be trained.

For the present authors these questions took on greater importance when the department of Clinical, Health and Personality Psychology of the University of Leiden, the Netherlands, decided to reconstruct the traditional clinical psychology training program into a clinical health psychology training program. In our efforts to develop such a program we found that most formalized training programs exist in the United States, whereas only a few have emerged in Western Europe. However, the mechanism for training psychologists in the United States is quite different from that which is seen in most other countries of the world. Virtually all training for psychologists in the US is at the Ph.D. level whereas Ph.D. training for psychologists in Europe is rare. The advantages and disadvantages of both systems are elaborated on more fully by Maes and Kittel (this issue) but with this distinction in mind, it is possible to understand the recommendation of the American Psychological Association's Division of Health Psychology which endorsed Ph.D. training in health psychology as the required entry level (Stone, 1983a).

A recent review of the extent and content of the range of programs offering training in health psychology in the US indicates that this training is provided by specialized Ph.D. programs in health psychology and by many clinical psychology Ph.D. training programs for work in health care settings, including applied research settings, clinical setttings, health education, and public health and health planning (Istvan and Hatton, 1987). But it is questionable that the American standard of Ph.D. training should or could be applied to settings in other countries. In countries where most psychologists—regardless of their specialization—are trained at the masters degree level, a different model may be needed.

But what *is* the status of training in Health Psychology in other countries? The results of a survey (described in detail later in this article) indicate that in several countries some courses are now offered in health psychology. Additionally, Maes and Kittel (this issue) identify six training programs in health psychology in Western Europe. Unfortunately, specific information about the content of these programs is not known to the present authors, because to our knowledge no published descriptions or comparisons exist. But this will likely come quickly as professional associations for health psychologists are now developing in several countries. These will surely spur the development of more comprehensive training programs for health psychologists in these areas and will lead to more collaboration and information sharing as well. Specific developments in this regard have already begun in Australia and are described by Oldenburg and Owen (this issue). These authors note that original efforts were modeled on the early developments in the United States, but these have now been modified to meet the specific health care needs in Australia.

Despite national differences several generic issues need to be addressed by training programs if they are to adequately prepare psychologists for work in health care. These issues are covered by the following recommendations that are abstracted from the Summary of Recommendations of the National Working Conference on Education and Training in Health Psychology (Stone, 1983b) and which guide the development of health psychology programs in the US:

—Health psychology should offer two major training options: scientist and professional.

—Institutions that engage in training must have sufficient breadth and depth of resources to ensure that students receive a comprehensive training that is not limited to one theoretical perspective or one methodology.

—Training should provide experience and course content stressing the role of diverse characteristics—cultural, ethnic, gender, life style, age, and so on—in both providers' and consumers' participation in the health system.

—Training should provide an integrated mixture of theory and practice including hands-on involvement in research under the direction of highly qualified mentors.

—Training should place strong emphasis on research methodology, including appropriate biostatistical methods in addition to the usual methods used by psychologists.

—Training should emphasize and provide the requisite skills for successful interdisciplinary collaboration.

—Training should engender an appreciation by trainees of the impact of the health psychologist on health care setting, patients, families, and so on.

—Training should provide instruction in ethical, legal, and professional issues.

—Training should provide instruction in health care organization and health care policy.

—Training should include appropriate training in assessment and intervention skills.

—Training for health psychologists who will provide direct health care services to individuals or groups will further require an internship of at least a year's duration in an organized interdisciplinary health service training program engaged in both psychological and physical health care.

—Internship mentors should predominantly include health psychologists who are themselves well qualified to practice professional health psychology, and effectively model the scientist/practitioner (pp. 15–17).

With these points in mind, the next section of this article will present the results of an international survey which was designed to elicit information about the availability and content of training in health psychology. It was hoped that the results of this survey would provide guidelines for establishing a more uniform standard of training for health psychologists thereby strengthening the development and status of this emerging field.

METHOD

Because of a lack of worldwide standardization of academic training and insufficient knowledge of the specific training situations in different countries, the questionnaire was designed using a combination of North American and European academic standards as outlined in *Table 1*. Countries included in the survey were selected on the basis that their cultural backgrounds and foundations of psychology were comparable. This meant the exclusion of countries in Asia, Latin America, and Africa. It meant the inclusion of New Zealand and Australia, whose cultural backgrounds were considered to be European in origin.

Table 1 Structure of academic training of psychologists in North America and Europe/South Pacific.[a]

Level	*North American*	*European*
Beginning university	4 years undergraduate training at college/university	2–3 years training at university in general psychology[c]
Intermediate university	2 years graduate training in psychology at university[b]	2–3 years training at university in specific psychological field[c]
Advanced university	3 years professional and research training in psychology at university[b]	in most cases not structurally supplied by university[d]
Only in some places:		4 years research training at university and/or: 4 years professional training at university

[a]South Pacific is meant to encompass New Zealand and Australia.
[b]In the U.S. these are frequently combined to form one Ph.D. program, rather than two discrete programs.
[c]In Europe beginning and intermediate university levels are mostly combined into one graduate training program.
[d]Advanced university training in Europe is rarely formalized although in some countries the development of research and professional training programs is in progress.

In designing the questionnaire, training at beginning university level and at intermediate university level was differentiated from training at advanced university level.†

As illustrated in *Table 1* the combination of the North American Bachelor's and Master's training can be compared with the European university training: both lead to a diploma of psychology in general. In contrast to North America, where the focus of graduate training is on psychology in general, the European graduate programs encompass two to three years of elementary education in general psychology and two to three years with an emphasis on special applications such as clinical and health psychology. In the last two to three years most programs request that students complete an internship in an applied clinical setting as well as a thesis based on empirical research.

The North American Ph.D. training can be compared with the European approach becoming a doctor or qualified clinical psychologist: both imply a specialization in research and/or practice after graduation in psychology. Unlike North America, in Europe, Australia, and New Zealand only some countries, and within these countries only some universities, have recently developed formalized doctoral research training programs. In most European countries a dissertation means a lengthy endeavour of empirical research and writing, completed by individuals who are very often already employed as university teachers/researchers, so they can work in close collaboration with their mentor or major professor. Although formalized professional training programs have just started or are planned in Great Britain, Belgium, and Holland, in most European countries the organization of professional training is very heterogeneous. Professional training programs are very often supplied as individual courses or workshops by private psychotherapeutic institutions or (divisions) of the national psychological association.

With these differences in mind, a semi-structured questionnaire was constructed and sent to psychologists who were considered knowledgeable about the situation of health psychology in their country. Because of the large international differences it was impossible to validate the questionnaire for all participating countries. This, together with the fact that completion of the questionnaire proved to be difficult for many respondents, sheds doubt on the accuracy of the thus gathered data. However, since most respondents gave additional information on the training situation in their country, major trends in the development of Health Psychology could be delineated and are worthwhile to mention.

Participants were chosen either because of their membership of the European Health Psychology Society, because they had published on health psychology subjects, or because they had been referred to by other experts in the field. Questionnaires were sent to the USA, Canada, Australia, New Zealand, Norway, Sweden, Finland, Denmark, Poland, German Democratic Republic, Czechoslovakia, Bulgaria, Hungary, Federal Republic of Germany, Austria, Italy, Switzerland, Spain, France, Belgium, the Netherlands, Great Britain and Northern Ireland.

† In the following all training programs taking place before graduation in psychology will be referred to as graduate training programs.

All training programs taking place after graduation and leading to a doctoral degree for which a scientific dissertation is needed will be referred to as doctoral training programs.

All training programs taking place after graduation and leading to a professional identification for which no scientific dissertation is needed will be referred to as professional training programs.

The questionnaire contained 40 items covering the following areas:

1) Prevalence of clinical and health psychology within the national health care systems.

2) Specialized training programs in health psychology compared to clinical psychology training programs.

3) Professional status of psychologists in health care.

RESULTS

Questionnaires were returned by all except those in Denmark, Poland, Bulgaria, and France.† As suggested by the respondent from Northern Ireland these data were combined with those from Great Britain to provide a summary picture of the United Kingdom. Several comments on the questionnaire revealed that the differences are very great. Because of these differences adequate responding to the questionnaire was often considered to be impossible and more than half of the respondents provided additional information by means of a letter, program-descriptions, articles and reports on the organisation of psychological training in general and clinical and health psychology in particular.

Prevalence of Clinical and Health Psychology within the National Health Care Systems

The *estimated ratios* of clinical and health psychologists combined to total populations reveal that the prevalence of clinical and health psychology varies considerably between countries. Great variations in educational levels and the fact that in many countries registers for clinical psychology are non-existent prohibit straightforward comparisons of these ratios and clear interpretations of differences.

High ratios (up to 1:5000) were reported for the Netherlands, Canada, USA, Norway, Australia, Finland, Federal Republic of Germany, and Belgium. *Intermediate ratios* (up to 1:10,000) were reported for Switzerland and Spain. *Low ratios* (over 1:10,000) were reported for Hungary, German Democratic Republic, United Kingdom, Czechoslovakia, and Austria. For Italy only the ratio of psychologists in general to the total population could be given (1:8800), and for New Zealand no figures were reported.

Compared to the number of clinical psychologists, who in most countries represent (more than) half of all psychologists, the numbers of health psychologists, if existent or known, are much smaller. Estimations range from 4 in Austria (i.e. 0.4% of all psychologists and 1.2% of all clinical psychologists) to 10,000 in the USA (10% of all psychologists and 14% of all clinical psychologists).

In most countries on which data were reported‡, higher percentages of Ph.D.'s

† We express our gratitude to Gertrud Bronneberg, Ruth Burckhardt, Kerry Chamberlain, Rocio Fernandez-Ballesteros, Arne Holte, Michael Murray, Pierre L.-J. Ritchie, Hans-Dieter Rosler, Lothar R. Schmidt, Lucio Sibilia, Jaroslav Sturma, Bako Tihamer, Maila Upanne, Jan Vinck, John Weinman, Beate Wimmer-Puchinger and Helen R. Winefield for their cooperation. Special thanks are directed toward John Weinman and Stan Maes for suggesting names of prominent health psychologists.

‡ No data were reported for Hungary, Finland, Spain, United Kingdom, Australia, Italy, German Democratic Republic, Czechoslovakia, and New Zealand.

were found for health psychologists than for clinical psychologists. Where in the USA and Canada doctoral training comprises both research and practice aspects, and is required to be registered as a clinical psychologist, in most other countries doctoral training focuses primarily on research. This may mean that in Europe health psychologists achieve higher academic standards than clinical psychologists.

Specialized Training Programs in Health Psychology Compared to Clinical Psychology Training Programs

Table 2 contains the number of clinical and health psychology training programs at graduate, professional and doctoral level for each participating country as well as the estimated amount of overlap between training in health and clinical psychology.

Combining respondents' additional information with the answers to the questionnaire it seems that true specialized training programs in health psychology exist only in the United States and Canada. In the US health psychology training is confined to the Ph.D.-level, in Canada it is also included in graduate programs. In Europe health psychology training at graduate level is mostly part of clinical psychology training *if* differentiation within the general psychology program exists. Differentiation in graduate training programs seems especially lacking in Eastern Europe. In the South Pacific no special training programs in health psychology exist. As in Europe health psychology is comprised within the clinical psychology programs. In New Zealand health psychology is also taught in teacher's training, community psychology, and medical psychology.

Table 2 Clinical and health psychology training programs according to level and overlapping areas.

Country	*Health PS. level*[a]	*N*[b]	*Clin. PS. level*[a]	*N*[b]	*% Overlap HP-CPprogr*	*% HP's trained in HP/CP*
USA	doct.	20	doct.	200	30–40%	10/90%
Canada	doct.	10	doct.	18	75%	80/90%
Norway	doct.	1	prof.	?	5–10%	0/100%
Finland	prof.	?	prof.	?	100%	unknown
German Democratic Republic	none		prof.	?	100%	0/100%
Czechoslovakia	none		prof.	?	100%	0/100%
Hungary	none		prof.	?	100%	0/100%
Federal Republic of Germany	grad.	5	grad.	30	50%	5/50%
Switzerland	prof. in progress[c]		prof.	5	unknown	0/100%
Austria	doct.	1	none		not applicable	100/0%
Italy	none		prof.	?	not applicable	unknown
Spain	doct.	2	doct.	5	20%	20/80%
Belgium	doct.	1	prof.	6	15%	0/40%
Holland	doct. in progress		prof. in progress		30–50%	5/100%
United Kingdom	doct. in progress		prof.	9	depending on program	0/35%
Australia	none		doct.	7	not applicable	unknown
New Zealand	none		prof.	?	not applicable	unknown

[a]Only the highest level is given (grad. = graduate, prof. = professional, doct. = doctoral).
[b]Number of programs reported; "?" means that no numbers were or could be given.
[c]"In progress" means that programs are being developed.

In most countries the university program takes 4 to 5 years. In the first 2–3 years general topics including methodology and research statistics are taught and in the remaining 2–3 years students choose one or two application areas in which specific courses and skills labs are taken, an internship is completed, a research study is carried out and a thesis is written.

The international comparison of health psychology training programs is complicated by the fact that graduate training in (health) psychology varies between universities within one country. In Italy, for example, Health Psychology is part of the curriculum in clinical psychology at the university of Padua and part of the medical training for physicians at the university of Rome. In Norway Health Psychology is provided by three universities in different ways: in Oslo it is included in the Medical Faculty and primarily given to medical students, in Trondheim it is part of clinical psychology and focusses on research, and very recently the University of Bergen has begun a new department of Health Psychology.

As expected, doctoral and professional training in Europe and the South Pacific is hardly comparable to the North American Ph.D. training. Formalized programs that combine practical and scientific professional training rarely exist. Doctoral training is mainly done by completing a lengthy dissertation on a subject of one's choice. Professional training is frequently provided by health care institutions and/or private or specialized psychotherapeutic associations. If specialized and time limited programs are mentioned they are of recent origin or in the process of planning. In general, this kind of specialization takes another 5 years. The disadvantages of this situation are vividly illustrated by the situation in Italy. There, no formal doctoral or professional training in clinical or health psychology exists. Most practicing psychologists acquire their knowledge and skills by following courses provided by private psychotherapeutic associations. In the absence of national standards, the quality of the different programs varies widely. Therefore, the identification of clinical or health psychology as a socially approved profession is impossible. In the German Democratic Republic and in Hungary postgraduate training of psychologists in health care takes place within the medical faculty. There is no differentiation from clinical psychology. In Hungary, the programs are dominated by psychotherapeutic training. It is a general impression that this overlap between clinical and health psychology is especially true for the East European countries and for Finland. Recent developments have been reported however which indicate that psychologists in these countries are increasingly consulted in cases where somatic conditions exist and where illness prevention and health promotion are desired. In the South Pacific no special doctoral training in health psychology exists. Although in New Zealand a graduate course in health psychology is planned, most psychology departments concentrate on traditional clinical psychology and all provide a clinical psychology Ph.D. program. In Australia Master's and Doctoral degrees are offered by so-called tertiary institutions and comprise a mixture of research-only and research-plus-coursework arrangements. There are seven doctoral programs in clinical and one in clinical neuropsychology. These programs presumably include health psychology topics since graduates find work in health settings in addition to the more traditional psychiatric settings.

The overlap between health and clinical psychology is evident when the content of the various programs is reviewed.

Table 3 shows the combined frequency for all countries for each of the subjects that were considered relevant for either specialized clinical or health psychology training

Table 3 Subjects covered in clinical and health psychology training programs over countries (N = 17).

Subject	*HP-programs*	*CP-programs*
Psychopathology	7	13
Psychodiagnostics	7	13
Neuropsychology	6	11
Assessment procedures	8	12
Risk behaviours	5	2
Research	8	12
Professional and ethical issues	6	8
Primary prevention	6	2
Relapse prevention	7	4
Rehabilitation	9	7
Public health	6	3
Clinical interventions	6	13

programs. Because of the international differences, graduate, professional, and doctoral programs were combined. As can be seen from these data, all topics are covered by health psychology programs as well as by clinical psychology programs. As expected, health psychology programs pay relatively more attention to risk behaviours, primary prevention, relapse prevention, rehabilitation, and public health. Further inspection of the data from Canada and the USA reveals that these subjects are only provided in doctoral health psychology training programs and not in doctoral clinical psychology training programs in these countries.

Considering the training situations outlined above the conclusion seems legitimate that European, Australian, and New Zealand health psychologists cannot (yet) clearly be differentiated from clinical psychologists by their training.

Professional Status of Psychologists in Health Care

With the exception of Italy, the German Democratic Republic, and New Zealand all participants reported the existence of a National Psychological Association (NPA) with a section or division for clinical psychology. Most NPA's, except the ones in Austria, Belgium, the Federal Republic of Germany, Switzerland, and Czechoslovakia, have also a section/division for health psychology.

Almost all countries have accreditation processes for training programs in general psychology; none of the countries has an accreditation process for health psychology training programs. Accreditation processes are carried out by the NPAs as well as by the governments. In Finland and the East European countries they are the sole responsibility of the government.

Licensing and registration procedures are available in less than half of the countries. They are lacking in Belgium, Italy, and Czechoslovakia; plans are in progress in the Federal Republic of Germany, the United Kingdom and Austria. No data were available for New Zealand, Hungary, the German Democratic Republic, and Australia. If a psychologist is registered or licensed, he/she can practice independently as far as the western countries are concerned. In Eastern Europe independent practice is unknown in the health care system. However, the allowance for independent practice does not imply direct reimbursement from the government and/or private health insurance companies. Governmental reimbursement does not hold for psychologists in Belgium, Canada, the Netherlands, Switzerland, Italy, Austria. Reimbursement from private insurance companies is only reported for Canada, the Federal Republic of Germany, Norway, Spain, and the US. In Australia and Holland it depends on the company's policies.

In general, psychologists have less professional status than medical doctors. They have less legal responsibilities, receive lower salaries, and are considered less powerful and/or professional by the general public. Some respondents therefore thought psychologists to be professionally isolated and discriminated against. Despite these "objective" differences, psychologists and medical doctors seem to collaborate well on a personal level. Competition for patients was considered a relatively minor problem especially in Europe, Australia, and New Zealand. The reason for this is, however, less fortunate than one might think. Since medical doctors are protected by a closed medical system and long established rules on financial and insurance procedures, they do not have to compete with psychologists. And at the moment, in most countries, psychologists are not powerful enough to change these long standing traditional boundaries, although some national psychological associations are beginning to address this issue.

DISCUSSION

The information outlined above has been gathered by means of an unvalidated questionnaire which many participants found rather difficult to complete correctly. This, of course, throws serious doubt on the accuracy of our data. Despite these methodological flaws, the qualitative material, which was spontaneously provided, together with the data from the questionnaire gave sufficient information for those interested in the development of Health Psychology in general and Health Psychology training in particular.

Although there exist great international differences in the organisation of the training of health psychologists, a general statement which can be made is that health psychology in Europe, Australia, and New Zealand is still in its infancy. Since health psychology on the whole is a rather new branch in psychology it can profit from internatinal collaboration in setting up appropriate training programs that represent international standards of qualification.

Presently, psychologists that can be called health psychologists were originally trained as clinical psychologists or as research psychologists. In Europe health psychologists more frequently have a doctoral degree than practising clinical psychologists. In order to maintain this relatively high scientific level among health psychologists and to incorporate clinical aspects it is advocated that future training programs encompass research training as well as practical professional training. In this way the scientific and practical base for health psychology as an independent discipline within psychology will be guaranteed.

It has been found that health psychology training programs overlap considerably with clinical psychology programs. For many components this overlap is justifiable and should be continued. On the other hand, true health psychological areas such as primary and secondary prevention, psychological applications in somatic conditions, and psycho-education could be better emphasized and specified whereas specific psychotherapeutic approaches could be left out of such programs. For the development of health psychology training programs in the future it is therefore recommended to consider the recommendations made by the National Working Conference on Education and Training in Health Psychology (Stone, 1983b) mentioned earlier in this article as well as the guidelines formulated by Singer (1987). These can be summarized as:

—Training in methodology is essential including statistics, experimental design, psychometrics, evaluations, meta-analyses, quasi-experimental procedures, and other techniques that can be used by research teams.

—Substantive knowledge in specific areas of health psychology is necessary.

—General health delivery systems and knowledge of specific organization structures is essential to the conduct of practice and research in health psychology.

—It is imperative that all health psychologists have both research and clinical skills (p. 117).

For a good understanding of these recommendations a more detailed discussion of some of these points seems in order:

1) Regardless of the location or level of training, the content and the design of training in health psychology should focus on the problems which are endemic to the health system in a given location. For instance, in most of the developed world, chronic illnesses and diseases such as coronary heart disease, cancer of all kinds, and accidents from a variety of causes, are now of primary importance. However, in the developing world the most important health problems are still those that are caused by micro-organisms, poor diet, and bad sanitary conditions, even though the previously mentioned disorders of the developed world are also prevalent. The health care system must address those disorders of primary importance in order to be effective and health psychologists must be trained to carry out the full range of professional activities which can benefit the health care system in their given locale. This includes research to determine the links between behaviors, the environment, and attitudes which influence health or illness, an awareness of the methods of educating the public and policy makers about how best to improve the health of citizens, and clinical intervention methods which will be both accepted and effective (Russo, 1985).

2) Because health is critical to all other aspects of life, health psychologists can contribute to the improvement of quality of life and health in a variety of ways. In addition to research and clinical intervention another less frequently discussed area is public health education as part of health prevention programs. Prevention programs are those which hold the most promise for reducing morbidity and mortality from the major causes of death and disability in the developed world: heart disease and cancer. Thus, health education programs designed to prevent teenagers from beginning the smoking habit, for example, can play a major role in the encouragement of healthier lifestyles and can make a significant difference in the future health of the world's population.

3) Health psychologists can also use their knowledge to influence government leaders and other influential policy makers about the important relationship between lifestyle, behaviors, emotional stress factors, and general health. However, health psychologists can only do this effectively if they are made aware of the importance

and appropriateness of such activities during their training programs. Involvement of health psychologists in these kinds of public education and political activities is a further reason for a strong science-based curriculum which lends credibility to the directions advocated by health psychologists (Singer, 1987).

4) Training programs should be designed to enhance the professional credibility and status of psychologists in health care. In order to accomplish this, they must be rigorous and based on sound knowledge, but must also stress the importance of acting within the boundaries of current knowledge. Health psychologists must also learn how to work with other professionals in the health care system, and to be familiar with the established language and norms of medical settings (Tapp, 1984). An essential part of the training should be carried out in interdisciplinary settings in order to allow for a greater collaboration between future health professionals and to contribute to the understanding of the appropriate role of each in the health care system. Concomitant with this is a need for health psychology training programs to incorporate a greater emphasis on topics such as medical terminology, psychopharmacology, and other topics previously thought to be outside the realm of psychologists (Stokes, Alexander, Lewis, Fischetti, and Rutledge, 1987).

5) Finally some recommendations can be made with regard to specific content areas. These content areas are generic to any training program in health psychology and should be included in the formulation of all such programs. A brief listing will suffice here: physiology, pharmacology, mechanisms of disease, behavioral influence and lifestyle effects on prevention of illness and promotion of health, health interventions, and epidemiology. And substantial information is needed on the mechanisms of illnesses such as coronary heart disease, cancer, asthma, diabetes mellitis, cystic fibrosis, epilepsy, and others on which the health psychologist can have an impact either in prevention or in terms of treatment compliance or psychological assistance to the patient and family (Russo, 1985; Swan, Piccione, and Anderson, 1980).

At the professional level health psychologists are poorly represented. This means that professional interests receive insufficient attention. Precisely the fact that health psychology is a new profession may provide the impetus for the development of professional organizations to promote and protect the occupational interests of health psychologists. It is therefore suggested that health psychologists organise themselves at national levels either by creating a division for health psychology within a national psychological association or by creating a national health psychological association itself. These national associations should exchange information, support and knowledge through the already established international health psychology societies.

References

Istvan, J. and Hatton, D. (1987). Curricula of graduate training programs in health psychology. In Stone, G., Weiss, S., Matarazzo, J., *et al.* (Eds.) *Health Psychology: A Discipline and a Profession*. Chicago: University of Chicago Press.

Russo, D. (1985). Clinical training in behavioral health psychology. *The Behavior Therapist*, **8**, 43–46.

Singer, J. (1987). Training for applied research in health psychology. In Stone, G., Weiss, S., Matarazzo, J., *et al.* (Eds.) *Health Psychology: A Discipline and a Profession*. Chicago: University of Chicago Press.

Stokes, D., Alexander, M., Lewis, J., Fischetti, L. and Rutledge, A. (1987). Difficulties in family practice residency training: Recommendations for training health psychologists in primary care settings. *Professional Psychologist*, **18**, 629–633.
Stone, G. (Ed.) (1983a). Proceedings of the National Working Conference on Education and Training in Health Psychology. *Health Psychology*, **2**, Supplement, Whole.
Stone, G. (1983b). Summary of recommendations. *Health Psychology*, **2**, Supplement, 15–18.
Swan, G., Piccione, A. and Anderson, D. (1980). Internship training in behavioral medicine: Program description, issues and guidelines. *Professional Psychology*, **11**, 339–346.
Tapp, J. (1984). Health psychology: an evolving discipline for psychologists. *Psychotherapy in Private Practice*, **2**, 49–64.

SECTION THREE

HEALTH PSYCHOLOGY TRAINING FOR OTHER HEALTH PROFESSIONALS

CHAPTER 11

TRAINING HEALTH PROFESSIONALS IN HEALTH PSYCHOLOGY

HAL SWERISSEN† and PETER FOREMAN

Department of Behavioural Health Sciences La Trobe University 625 Swanston Street Carlton, Victoria 3053 Australia

Health psychology has become a significant, if variable component of the academic curriculum for allied health professionals. This article reviews the relevance of training in health psychology for allied health professionals and some of the more controversial issues which have emerged, before suggesting a framework for future developments.

INTRODUCTION

Health professions, such as nursing, physiotherapy, occupational therapy, speech pathology, and podiatry (chiropody) have traditionally provided services at the direction of medical practitioners and as such they were characterized as an adjunct to medicine. Overwhelmingly employing women, often working part time, these allied health or paramedical professionals, have conducted the bulk of the day to day health service delivery. In the past, relatively poorly paid and subject to rigid hierarchies dominated by medicine, they have had only limited autonomy over their own roles. Generally an apprenticeship training model, conducted in the setting in which they worked, such as the hospital, reinforced these arrangements (Cosh, 1971; Sims, 1967).

More recently there have been significant changes in the philosophy, organization and training of the allied health professions. Employment in these professions has grown dramatically since the 1940s, reflecting the general growth in health expenditure. In Australia, for example the number of people per 100,000 working in health services grew at 2.5% per year between 1974 and 1984. Nursing made up the vast majority of this growth, with nearly six fold more nurses than medical practitioners employed in the health sector. The remaining health professionals comprised about one and half times as many people as the number of medical practitioners (Australian Institute of Health 1988).

As part of this growth, roles and responsibilities have also expanded and become more complex. Clearly, this is partly due to the introduction of increasingly more sophisticated technology into hospital settings. However, broader policy developments affecting the health system have also been important. Most notably, the impact of the rising costs of health care, the trend toward community based

†To whom correspondence should be addressed.

services, the demands for services to be responsive to the social and psychological context in which they are delivered, and the developing emphasis on disease prevention and health promotion (Pelligrino, 1974). As a result, more health professionals have found themselves working in non-hospital settings and also in multidisciplinary teams with complex and shifting roles and responsibilities.

In conjuction with these broad changes to their duties and responsibilities, not surprisingly, professions such as nursing, physiotherapy and occupational therapy have pursued their own professional development in an attempt to assert independence over their work and gain greater status and remuneration. Inevitably, that has placed stress on the relationship between allied health professions and medicine. In response to increasing complexity and diversity in their work and in the quest for the expansion of professional autonomy, allied health professionals have sought and been successful in relocating their training from field settings, like hospitals to universities and colleges (Gardener and McCoppin 1989).

The move from hospital based, apprentice-type practitioner training for groups such as occupational therapists, physiotherapists and nurses began in the United States in the 1950s, in Canada in the early 1960s and Australia in the late 1960s (Sawner, 1971; Peak, 1971). In the United Kingdom the tranistion is still underway as it is in Australia in the case of nurse education. The move into mainstream higher education was accompanied by significant changes to the training curricula which lead to, in most cases, the introduction of substantial academic studies, including psychology and other behavioural sciences.

Health psychology curriculum development

Our own institution provides a good example of the academic evolution of psychology training for the allied health professions. During the triennium 1972–1975 our diploma courses in Physiotherapy, Occupational Therapy and Communication Disorders (Speech Therapy) were restructured and redeveloped as bachelors degrees in Applied Science and a Department of Behavioural Sciences was established with the specific brief of providing all behavioural science teaching in the allied health programs. One consequence of these developments was a notable increase in the amount of behavioural sciences in the allied health curricula. For example, by 1976 the new physiotherapy degree included four and a half hours per week of behavioural science content in first year, four hours per week in second year and lesser but still significant amounts in the remaining terms. This represented an increase in behavioural sciences content of approximately one hundred percent compared to the earlier diploma course. Psychology comprised the largest component of the behavioural science content.

By and large, as was the case in our own program, psychology training in college and university based courses for allied health professionals has fallen into three curriculum areas: general psychology, research methods and interpersonal processes or counselling. In the absence of curricula designed specifically for the health sciences, reflected in the paucity of relevant text books, psychology educators have been faced with a choice of basing their teaching on the more established curricula developed for either undergraduate psychology or medical students. Inevitably content, teaching hours, and teaching approaches have been widely divergent. Probably the most common model has been for psychologists to be employed in an adjunct role to conduct 'service' teaching, either as a member of a professional department or as part of a psychology unit providing teaching to a number of professional departments.

It is tempting to assume that psychology constitutes a basic science for the practice of allied health professionals in the same way as physiology is assumed to be a basic science for medicine. Developing the curriculum might then be thought of as selecting relevant theory and content from general psychology, for example, learning and cognition, developmental psychology and so on, and teaching these in a health context. Unfortunately such an assumption depends on there being a systematic link, based on scientific research, between the development of practice for allied health professionals and psychological theory.

Paradoxically, psychological theory and practice has influenced a number of assessment and intervention strategies employed in professions such as physiotherapy, speech pathology and occupational therapy and a number of researchers in these professions have held psychology qualifications. Productive research programs between psychology and the allied health professions continue to flourish and psychologists regularly contribute to the professional literature in these areas. But these influences have rarely been been directly reflected in curriculum development for allied health courses.

To some extent those who initially developed the psychology curriculum for the allied health professions, responded to prevailing liberal education ideology which emphasised the values of intellectual breadth and scholarship and the behavioural sciences, including psychology, were seen as very appropriate in this context. However the specific educational rational underlying the increase in behavioural science content in curricula for allied health professionals was frequently poorly defined and, we would now argue, based on limited assumptions about the role of the behavioural sciences, and psychology in particular, in health care. For example the bahavioural sciences with their focus on the psychosocial dimensions of behaviour have been justified and promoted within allied health education on the grounds that they provide a perspective for understanding illness and illness management that is complementary to the medical-model thinking within the allied health groups. In a similar vein it has been argued that psychology programs in allied health curricula encourage the 'whole' person view of patient care and that psychology, with its stress on the individual and individual-environment interactions, could counterbalance the tendency of core professional studies to focus on diseases and disabilities rather than people (Wexler, 1976).

Despite the potential for successful collaboration between psychologists and allied health professionals, the psychology curriculum for allied health professionals remained relatively insensitive to the needs of the allied health professions. Unfortunately, where a 'psychology centred' philosophy is adopted and there is little attempt to integrate the health psychology curriculum with the actual problems and practice concerning allied health professionals, it is unlikely that allied health students will see the relevance of the curriculum to their professional development. A problem which is further exacerbated where there are few models of joint research programs or professional collaboration between psychology and allied health staff.

Rather than basing curriculum development on the structure traditional for psychology courses, it may be more fruitful for the health psychology curriculum to reflect a health focus. This raises some definitional issues about 'health'. In that respect, as Diekstra notes elsewhere in this volume, health is now increasingly viewed in a social context and the 'medical model' is coming under strong pressure from a biopsychosocial model (e.g. Engel 1977) set within a health continuum, which includes health promotion, and primary, secondary, and tertiary prevention of disease and injury. Such an approach is broadly consistent with the position taken by the World Health Organization and a social approach to health now has wide credibility as reflected by its increasing emphasis in the health policies of the OECD nations. Arguably, psychology applied to heath issues within such a health framework has more to offer health science students because it is more likely to demonstrate the relevance of psychological theory and practice directly to issues that concern them in a framework they can readily understand.

Ultimately, the degree to which the health psychology curriculum has a health or psychology focus and the extent to which it is concerned with practice, depends on the overall structure and organization of the curriculum. Where a generalist, liberal arts and sciences introduction to allied health courses is emphasized there is more scope for an explicitly psychological orientation. On the other hand, those courses which are more exclusively oriented to professional training are likely to require psychology to demonstrate its relevance more explicitly. Inevitably context specific factors will influence curriculum philosophy and development. Of course many of these issues reoccur in other professional courses where psychology programs have been developed for non-psychologists such as medicine and primary and secondary education.

VOCATIONAL RELEVANCE

What was largely missing from the psychology curriculum for the allied health sciences debate -which was characteristic of the Australian situation at least in the 1970s – was the recognition that psychological techniques and theories have a more direct contribution to make to the actual vocational behaviour of allied health workers as they engage in their work of preventing and ameliorating the effects of illness, injury or disability and promoting and maintaining health.

Moreover, simply justifying psychology in terms of its humanizing or enriching educational function placed it in a purely ancillary role in the education of health professionals. The contributions of psychology were limited to 'rounding off' the education of these students and filling in the gaps and cracks that appeared in professional studies curricula under the strain of coping with complex health settings and broader and different roles for health professionals. Apart from perhaps communication and counselling skills, there was little emphasis on the role psychology might play in improving practice.

Over time psychology curricula for the health sciences have become more vocationally relevant in response to a numbver of convergent trends. Most important perhaps is that psychologists over the last decade at least have developed a body of research and applied knowledge concerned with the application of psychology to health problems; that is the area broadly defined as health psychology. Many of the findings and intervention strategies arising from health psychology research in areas such as the cognitive and behavioural determinants of physical health and disease, behavioural diagnostic techniques, pain and its management, adherence, and behavioural contributions in the the treatment and rehabilitation of physical disorders are directly relevant to the vocational skills of many allied health professionals.

As well, the role of allied health practitioners have expanded and evolved over the last decade to encompass a broader range of client populations, therapeutic and preventive activities, they have become disenchanted with biomedical models. The impact of current concerns with, for example, health promotion and the prevention of illness and injury, rehabilitation following work injury, normalisation and deinstitutionalization and the aged population and the reflection of these concerns in economic and legislative changes has had a major impact on the activities of many of the allied health professions (e.g. White, 1986; Allen, Graham, Hiep & Tonkin, 1988; Madill, Brintnell & Stewin, 1989; Bunker, Parcel, Phillips & Simons-Morton, 1986).

The implications of these role expansions for education and training have also been widely acknowledged. For example, in the United States the National Commission on Allied Health Education (1980) specifically recommended that all allied health education programs include the study of illness prevention and health promotion methods and noted that allied health education would be required to move away from the then current emphasis on human biology and health care organisation and become more concerned with the influence of the social and physical environment and individual life-style on health outcomes. As a consequence more weight has been placed on the inclusion of the behavioural sciences in the core curricula for these professions.

Finally, direct feedback from students and other allied health academics have also had an impact. Psychologists teaching in allied health faculities realised that so long as their offerings were seen as peripheral to the major vocational activities of their students and did not directly impinge on their clinical experiences then health psychology courses would be treated as marginal in importance. All of these pressures have influenced the trend for psychology teaching for allied health professionals to become more health and vocation oriented.

CONTRADICTIONS AND ISSUES

However it would be naive to assume that a match between what health psychologists claim they can offer and the apparent skill requirements of allied health groups will ensure that relevant health psychology skills will be readily and effectively included in initial allied health education programs. With the notable exception of counselling or communication skills teaching, which now appears to be almost universally included in allied health science curricula (e.g., Schultz, Wellard & Swerissen 1988), the picture is very mixed. A recent survey of psychology teaching in British physiotherapy schools showed a wide range of psychology offerings including traditional topics of memory, personality and so forth, a small number of hours (less than two on average) devoted to any one topic and a clear preference for the use of lectures (Baddely & Bithell, 1989). This relative lack of enthusiasm for what health psychology can offer in the training of allied health professional may simply reflect the newness of the field, but it is likely that more fundamental issues about the acceptance of health psychology as a core area of study are at stake.

Most importantly, the incorporation of health psychology skills and procedures into the training programs for the allied health occupations, and thus into the vocational practices of these health workers, raises difficult issues of professional autonomy and professional overlap as well as problems of curriculum design. Gaining professional autonomy is a central preoccupation of most of the allied health occupations (Gardner & McCoppin, 1989). The key dimension of professionalism is autonomy or control over the direction of ones work and an important characteristic of a profession is the possession of an exclusive body of knowledge and skills (Friedson, 1984). Most allied health professionals have placed emphasis on the development of specific assessment and intervention practices in which they are seen to have expertise and which they control. For example, the development of nursing diagnoses, the use of heat therapy and transcutaneous stimulation by physiotherapists, the development of activities of daily living (ADL) measures by occupational therapists and so on. The acceptance of theories and procedures derived from health psychology as part of the core training curriculum can be perceived as threat to a group trying to establish itself as an independent profession with an exclusive body of knowledge and skills.

A related issue concerns the amount and type of teaching time required to adequately develop proficiency in practical psychological methods. Training allied health students in the application of psychological methods requires significant time in what are typically very packed curricula and often necessitates a re-ordering of traditional curriculum priorities. By way of illustration, McKenzie & Chinnery (1988) examined the extent to which physiotherapy trainees used behavioural techniques in the management of chronic back pain after taking a twenty hour course on the use of such techniques. The authors attributed the less than optimal utilization rate of techniques such as shaping, reinforcement and contracting, to lack of practise, lack of appropriate role models in the clinical environment, and inadequate depth of knowledge. Similarly Fisher, Nurse and Kennedy (1989) showed that nurses who under took a brief course in behavioural techniques for pain management demonstrated an increased knowledge of behavioural principles, but no changes in their ability to specify behavioural problems. These examples illustrate the difficulty of adequately teaching health psychology techniques to those whose primary orientation is to another discipline.

Problems of depth of knowledge, limited access to clinical training settings and lack of appropriate role models should make psychologists wary of devaluing their skills through inadequate teaching of them to other health practitioners. A further difficulty arises from the desirability of a close and mutually influencing nexus between intervention practices and research. Psychologists are generally educated in a culture where this interaction is stressed. Witness the emphasis on the scientist-practitioner model in the literature on both clinical and health psychology practice. This is not currently the case, or at least nor to the same extent, for other health related occupations.

Of course psychologists are not indifferent to professional concerns; for us the question becomes, to what extent and under what conditions should psychologists train others to practice applied psychology? As Stachnik (1980) noted in his seminal article wherein he outlined the new direction for psychologists in health care, if psychologists do not get into the area of changing health related behaviours others will, Yet, while there is little doubt that psychology has contributed to our understanding and ability to prevent and ameliorate health problems, the extent to which health psychology can be thought of as a separate discipline or profession remains hotly disputed within psychology (e.g. Matarazzo, 1987). Moreover, it is extremely unlikely that sufficient numbers of health psychologists will be trained and employed in health settings to adequately apply those health psychology models and strategies which have been developed to materially affect the quality and succes of health services and programs.

IMPLICATIONS

These issues constitute a challenge for the psychologist- educator but they also highlight more general concerns about the place and role of health psychology vis-a-vis other professions in the delivery of effective health care. While psychologists would appear to have developed very relevant skills and knowledge; given the relatively high ratio of allied health professionals to health psychologists, it is the allied health professionals who are more likely than psychologists to be in a position to employ these skills. Undoubtedly, educating allied health professionals in health psychology, particularly insofar as specific skills are taught, to some extent involves 'giving psychology away', and it must therefore erode health psychology's claims to exclusive expertise. Nevertheless, it is arguable, despite concerns about professional demarcation and the quality of health psychology training provided to allied health professionals, that educating them in the use of these skills remains one of the few strategies, apart from conducting and disseminating research, that health psychology has to ensure it has a widespread impact on health outcomes.

In the light of these concerns, developing an appropriate psychology curriculum for allied health science education constitutes a difficult task for both the psychologist and the allied health professional. At one level it is important to avoid marginalizing health psychology so that it does not become an introduction on 'how humans behave', while remaining mindful of not falling into the trap of trying to make inadequately trained health psychologists out allied health trainees. At the same time the real contribution of health psychology to the understanding of the development and treatment of conditions addressed by allied health professions must be communicated in the interests of effective health care delivery.

Given all these constraints, what might a health psychology curriculum for allied health professionals include? Firstly, one could continue to adopt a traditional liberal-arts philosophy and thereby ensure allied health students undertake psychology courses very similar to those taken by psychology students. For a range of reasons, which we have outlined above, that is not our preferred approach. Instead, our view is that the curriculum might be thought of as comprising two strands. First health psychology training for health professionals should ensure that health professionals develop a knowledge of the role behavioural and psychological factors play in the development and treatment of, and recovery from both general and specific illness and injury conditions which are relevant to the clinical populations, health problems and intervention settings of concern to a particular allied health group. Content areas might include perceptions of health and health beliefs throughout the lifespan; psychological and social factors in the development and maintenance of behavioural health risks such as tobacco use, overeating and alcohol abuse; the role of social support in the development and recovery from disease; the interaction between physiological; psychological and social factors in stress and pain; and psychological reactions to illness; hospitalization, disability and death.

In this strand the curriculum would ensure that students are able to critically analyze health issues from a psychological perspective. In that respect, the health psychology curriculum could be characterized as health focussed and it is to be hoped that in future, following the experience of psychology in relation to medicine, health psychology text books and other materials for the health sciences which are responsive to this philosophy will become available. However, while the role of research and inquiry would be emphasized and implications for practice noted, within this strand, vocationally relevant skills would not be taught directly. These would form the primary focus for the second strand of the curriculum.

In the second strand, health psychology training should teach vocationally relevant skills which can be readily assimilated into the role of the allied health professional, are relatively independent of an extended knowledge base in psychology, and do not require continual supervision by a psychologist in order to be performed effectively. In this respect, the inclusion of research and communication skills in the curriculum is relatively well accepted, although it might be noted that while they are usually taught to health professionals by psychologists, these skills are thought of as generic (at least within the Australian context) and are therefore not necessarily identifed with psychology. Other skills such as program planning and evaluation, task analysis and case management, and strategies to ensure adherence with treatment regimes might also fall into this category.

Ideally, of course the knowledge base of health psychology and the vocationally relevant skills derived from it would be taught in an integrated program. We have separated these strands for two reasons. First, pragmatically, it is not always possible to fully include both components in the curriculum. For example, aspects may be resisted by allied health educators because they are seen as irrelevant or infringing on their professional expertise. Or there may simply be insufficient time and resources. Second, they require different teaching approaches. While health psychology theory and research can be taught within the classroom in lecture, seminar and tutorial formats, vocational skills are more likely to require a competency based approach which includes practice and supervision in applied or psuedo-applied settings. As such, they are more intensive and require health psychology educators who have relevant applied skills.

Finally, it is obvious that curriculum philosophy and content have implications for the relationships between health psychology and allied health educators. It seems possible, but not entirely satisfactory, for health psychology educators who teach allied health students to have a relatively separate academic existence from that of allied health educators and still successfully teach the first strand of the health psychology curriculum. However, it is difficult to see health psychology educators successfully teaching vocationally relevant skills and influencing the *practice* of allied health professionals without them having constructive and collaborative relationships with their allied health colleagues. In a sense the relationship between health psychologists and allied health professionals involved in training might constitute a potential third strand of the curriculum strategy whereby health psychologists and allied health professionals jointly develop specific research and intervention programs which influence health care through the training of future health professionals. It is to be hoped that more collaborative activity of this nature occurs in the future.

References

Australian Institute of Health (1988). *Australia's health*, Canberra: Australian Government.

Allen, G., Graham, J., Hiep, M. and Tonkin, M. J. (1988). Occupational therapy 1981–1986: Trends and implications. *Australian Occupational Therapy Journal*, **35,** 155–164.

Baddely, H. and Bithell, C. (1989). Psychology in the physiotherapy curriculum. *Physiotherapy*, **75,** 17–21.

Bunker, J. J. F., Parcel, G. S., Phillips, B. V. and Simons-Morton, D. (1986). Curriculum implications of health promotion and disease prevention in allied health education. *Journal of Allied Health*, **15**(4), 339–357.

Cosh, P. (1971). The challenge of physiotherapy education in Australia. *The Australian Journal of Physiotherapy*, **17**(4), 113–118.

Engel, G. (1977). The need for a new medical model: The challenge to biomedicine.*Science*, **196,** 129–136.

Fisher, K., Nurse, M. and Kennedy, P. (1989) Teaching nurses behavioural methods for pain management: A pilot study. *Behavioural Psychotherapy*, **17**(3), 283–289.

Friedson, E. (1984). Dominant professions, bureaucracy and client services. In Y. Hasenfield and R. A.

English (Eds.). *Human service organizations*, University of Michigan Press, Ann Arbor.
Gardner, H. and McCoppin, B. (1989). Emerging militancy? The politicisation of Australian allied health professionals. In H. Gardner (Ed.). *The politics of health: The Australian experience*, Churchill Livingstone, Melbourne.
McKenzie, W. C. and Chinnery, D. L. (1988). Educational needs of health professions in treatment of low back pain. *Australian Journal of Physiotherapy*, **34**(1).
Madill, H., Brintnell, S. and Stewin, I. (1989). Professional literature: One view of a national perspective. Australian *Occupational Therapy Journal*, **36**(3), 110–119.
Matarazzo, J. D. (1987). Challenges and opportunities in training health psychologists. In G. C. Stone, S. M. Weiss, J. D. Matarazzo, N. E. Miller, J. Rodin, C. D. Belar, M. J. Follick and J. E. Singer (Eds.). *Health psychology: A discipline and a profession*, Chicago: University of Chicago Press.
Peak, L. N. (1971). Occupational therapy, nursing and physiotherapy. *Archives of Physical Medicine and Rehabilitation*, **52**(9), 406–498.
Pelligrino, E. D. (1974). Preventive health care and the allied health professions. In J. Hamburg (Ed.). *Review of allied health education*: 1. Kentucky: University of Kentucky Press.
Sawner, K. A. (1971). Physiotherapy, medicine and occupational therapy. *Archives of Physical Medicine and Rehabilitation*, **52**(9), 408–410.
Schultz, C. L., Wellard, R. and Swerissen, H. (1988). Communication and interpersonal helping skills: An essential component of physiotherapy education? *Australian Journal of Physiotherapy*, **34**(2), 75–80.
Sims, G. E. (1967). Sylvia Docker lecture: Occupational Therapy in Australia, the formative years. *Australian Occupational Therapy Journal*, **14**(1), 29–44.
Stachnik, T. J. (1980). Priorities for psychologists in medical education and health care delivery. *American Psychologist*, **35,** 8–15.
The National Commission on Allied Health Education. (1980). *The future of allied health education*. San Francisco: Jossey-Bass Publishers.
Wexler, M. (1976). The behavioural sciences in medical education: A review from psychology. *American Psychologist*, **36,** 275–283.
White, V. K. (1986). Promoting health and wellness: A theme for the eighties. *Australian Occupational Therapy Journal*, **40**(11), 743–748.

CHAPTER 12

HEALTH PSYCHOLOGY FOR MEDICAL STUDENTS

HELEN R. WINEFIELD

Dept. Psychiatry, University of Adelaide, GPO Box 498, Adelaide, Australia 5001

This paper discusses a number of important issues associated with the teaching of health psychology to medical students. The first section focuses on what medical students need to learn about the field. It is argued that students should understand the scientific basis and methods of psychology as well as the psychological theories and findings that relate to health behaviour and the delivery of health care and the psychological skills that can be used in clinical practice. Furthermore they need to be aquainted with the specialist skills of health psychologists, as future fellow health professionals. The teaching should be given by health psychologists who are aware of and sympathetic to key issues and concepts in medicine and should include basic and applied areas of psychology. In the long term, successful teaching should result in a growing mutual respect between health psychology and medicine and thus serve to bring substantial benefits to both disciplines.

INTRODUCTION

Because medical practitioners need to comfort, persuade and educate in the course of improving health, a knowledge base in the science of human behaviour is an essential component of their training. The emergent subject of health psychology has much to offer medical education, and much to gain from participating in it. This chapter will, after referring to the history and nature of health psychology, be organized around the following questions:

1) what do medical students need to know about health psychology?
2) how is health psychology best taught to medical students?
3) what are the short- and long-term consequences of health psychology being included in medical education?

As health psychology is a relatively new intellectual discipline, many discussions begin with efforts to define it. Stone (1990, p. 7) takes the wide view that health psychology "encompasses any scientific or professional application of psychological concepts or methods to any problem arising in the health system". Health psychology is a body of knowledge, while the term behavioural medicine refers more specifically to the application of behavioural techniques to achieve medical goals. Taylor (1990) identifies some characteristics which distinguish health psychology from medicine: the former looks for broad principles of human behaviour such as the connection between health and feelings of control, whereas medicine is disease-focussed; health psychologists work to keep people out of the health care system, and are concerned to monitor changing patterns of illness and disease and their implications. Taylor reviews a large number of applications of psychological knowledge to health and illness, and notes a movement of health psychologists from peripheral to central roles in the health enterprise.

HEALTH PSYCHOLOGY IN THE MEDICAL CURRICULUM: WHAT DO STUDENTS NEED TO LEARN?

Courses taught by psychologists have been introduced into medical curricula all over the world in the last two decades. They vary in their titles, with Behavioural Science and Medical Psychology being favourites, in the academic departments which teach them, and in their timing within the medical course, but the content is predominantly health psychology in the terms of Stone's definition cited above. While a variety of considerations originally prompted the introduction of such courses, the field is now sufficiently mature to consider exactly what medical graduates need to know about health psychology. I suggest that they need to know that a science of human behaviour exists, what methods of enquiry and knowledge it incorporates, and how it applies to medical practice, both as part of every doctor's understanding and skills, and as an field of specialist expertise.

1) *There are scientific techniques applicable to the understanding of human behaviour, and psychologists are the professionals who develop and use them.*

The principles of enquiry and knowledge accumulation which have proven so powerful in the the physical and biological sciences are not only relevant but also fruitful when applied to human behaviour. As most incoming medical students have no experience of social science at school, they sometimes tend to regard human behaviour in its wonderful complexity as being beyond the reach of rational explanation or study. Such views leave them prey to irrational explanations and beliefs. Without claiming that psychology is fully rational or has discovered precisely how to formulate and explore human behaviour in reliably scientific way, we can point to a basic respect for data-gathering and hypothesis-testing, with associated concern for standardized measurements, statistical probability, and control groups.

The principles of research design and methodology which are taught as part of health psychology, can of course be applied also to the evaluation of claims in other fields such as new pharmocological, procedural and technological discoveries.

2) *Psychological concepts, theories, and empirical findings are directly relevant to human health and illness and to the delivery of health care.*

Current psychological knowledge provides our best available tool for systematically understanding people and predicting and modifying their behaviour. While some of the received wisdom of today may lose ground during the student's professional career if better theories and models win acceptance, psychological study has revealed much about human thought, emotional reactions, personal development through life, the determinants of individual and group behaviour and correspondingly how to change them, individual differences and their measurement, coping with threatening circumstances, and the relations between mind and body. Roles, attitude change, group dynamics, team-work, and the workings of large institutions, are studied by health psychologists with a social rather than individual orientation. Quantitative research by psychologists, some in collaboration with other basic or applied scientists or medical practitioners, is proceeding with enthusiasm and offers hope of continuous knowledge gains. Which of us, given a choice of doctors equally knowledgeable about physiology and pharmocology, would not prefer to be treated by the one also knowledgeable about human behaviour and emotions?

3) *Psychological knowledge and techniques are useful for medical practitioners to employ routinely in their own practice.*

Practitioners are better equipped to understand the behaviour of their patients, colleagues, and indeed themselves, when they understand aspects of human adjustment including: the value of a sense of personal control, the role of attachments and social supports, pain perception and expression, the benefits and methods of constructive stress management, how illness behaviour habits are acquired, and what challenges and developmental tasks face people of different age groups. Professional efficacy is therefore likely to be enhanced and job strain decreased.

Diekstra (1990) lists the kinds of primary health care problem which call for psychological knowledge and skills: problems of anxiety and stress, habit disorders, educational and occupational difficulties or decisions, interpersonal-social-marital problems, and adjustment to physical illness and other significant life events. The strong emphasis in primary health care on education, prevention, and health promotion makes it all the more important that doctors grasp the principles of learning and behaviour change.

While the fore-going are all problems experienced by patients, one might add that problems in the delivery of health care have also been researched by psychologists. Interpersonal communication and the development of the helping relationship within medicine has been subjected to controlled empirical study, and the application of findings to medicine is vital for the face to face encounter which is the heart of healing. Even when the patient is unconscious, dealing with relatives, colleagues, and the doctor's own affective responses will all be enhanced by systematic understanding of these process aspects of care.

4) *Specialist health psychologists are available to take referrals of patients with problems beyond the doctor's clinical competence.*

Students need to know that some psychologists specialize in work of potential value to health care professionals - for example they work to change the health-related behaviours (including beliefs, emotional responses and overt behaviours) of individuals, groups, or whole communities. Stress management, alcohol and tobacco use, sexual and relationship difficulties, family violence, depression, rehabilitation, tension headaches – the lists of possible referral symptoms are long and familiar; what the clinical health psychologist has to offer is skills based on scientific research which is impressive and rapidly expanding.

Doctors in training need to understand the mechanisms and the likely outcomes of referring patients to specialist health psychologists for help with patient problems beyond the medical practitioner's own capacity to help, with that line being drawn at different places for different doctors depending on interests, study opportunities, and local referral options. It will probably be advisable to clarify differences between different varieties of psychologist, and between psychologists and other professionals such as psychiatrists and social workers.

HOW CAN HEALTH PSYCHOLOGY BEST BE TAUGHT TO MEDICAL STUDENTS?

Having outlined above the basic content of health psychology training for medical students, I now offer some comments about strategies for achieving this learning.

Pre clinical health psychology courses vary in the extent to which they seek to equip students with broad understanding of psychological principles, versus concentrating on the application of psychological knowledge to medically-relevant problems (Weinman, 1989). The topics in the latter kind of course tend to sound more interesting to students (e.g. sexuality, death, stress, child abuse, interviewing) than in the former (e.g. psychological development, emotion, attitude and behaviour change); no controlled trial of long-term retention and critical application of course materials in the two approaches has been carried out where both have equal weight in class-time and in student assessment. Ideally, there is reconciliation rather than opposition of these two approaches so that these very capable students are motivated to master the subject intellectually because they see its relevance to their chosen career in medical practice.

At the clinical and postgraduate levels of medical training, an applied focus is appropriate and congruent; educational input here has moved from the lecture theatre to the ward and clinic, following an apprenticeship model which has been accepted into other professional disciplines. The double goals of gaining student attention in the short-term, and of teaching them a life-long sympathetic and well-informed awareness of health psychology, pose dilemnas initially for instructors, but these must be resolved. Supportive discussion with colleagues in similar positions, through national organizations of health psychologists, is valuable. Feedback from students and medical school colleagues is essential, although the latter can be difficult to obtain.

Teaching Personnel

Who should do the teaching? Engel (1982, p. 805) argued that the "biopsychosocial" model should be taught by "physicians whose scientific model is biopsychosocial and who exemplify, in their everyday work, expertise in the psychosocial dimensions of their particular area of practice". He argued that psychiatrists alone could not effect acceptance of this holistic model because they are "not part of the mainstream of medicine". How much truer then, for psychologists, who have never even undergone the bond-forming traumas of medical training. It is vital for the success of health psychology training of medical students, that the subject matter should be perceived as an integral tool used by senior medical consultants. Active involvement by doctors in the health psychology teaching program at every level is therefore very desirable.

Psychologists must constantly decentre from their own cognitive framework in order to make clear the links between areas of psychological knowledge and the applications to clinical medicine (Winefield, 1981). Because students especially beginners may have vague or incorrect expectations of what medical care involves, they need information about that as well as about health psychology, in order to perceive the relevance of the latter. Students should be aware, to take simple examples, of the high frequency of patient noncompliance with medical intructions and of symptoms presented to doctors which have no discernible somatic cause, or which have directly behavioural causes. Thus teachers need to know about the process and realities of delivering medical care, as well as about the psychological principles which apply, so that they can relate the two clearly for students. The health psychologist teachers therefore must become familiar with some medical terminology and customs (Belar, 1990; Methorst, Jansen & Kerkhof, 1990).

The community's attitude to medical practitioners may best be characterized as ambivalent. Individual patients usually claim to be very satisfied with their care, but at the same time, negative comments concern doctor's power, income, cautiousness about information-giving, and failure to cure. Treatment mistakes and cases of professional malpractice are given media publicity as well as the "miracle" drugs and new techniques. The hostility to medicine of those disappointed that doctors cannot fix all health problems, is something which health psychologists must not unthinkingly convey. Teaching which is perceived as "anti-doctor" by the medical students will be dismissed by them and will indeed have counter-productive effects. Thus health psychology teachers must be seen to be sympathetic to the difficulties and trials of medical practice, and to be respected by the medically-qualified members of the Faculty.

Teaching Strategies

As suggested above, teaching strategies need to be congruent with the learning tasks of students at different stages of their medical course. Before patient contact begins, practical projects seem to be a particularly valuable supplement to the standard lectures and small-group tutorials. They demonstrate psychological concepts and skills to students concretely, and thus increase their memorability. Nonparticipant observations of medical settings provide rich opportunities for students to experience the helpfulness of a psychological framework (Peay, 1977); surveys of public opinion on health-relevant topics have a double value; likewise field studies with a developmental orientation give opportunities for learning about information-gathering as well as about childhood and parenthood (Winefield, 1990). These of course need to be appropriate to the level of student medical knowledge at the time. First-year students in the British/Australian system know negligible medicine, and therefore may have unrealistic ideas about what doctors do and therefore, about what it is necessary to learn.

This problem-oriented, "hands on" approach can also be applied to the task of learning to be a critical consumer of the research literature. Analyses of the design and methodology of published reports facilitates student confidence in being able to evaluate claims and continue self-directed learning life-long: goals acclaimed in successive reviews of medical education (Doherty, 1988; General Medical Council, 1987).

Health psychology training for medical students must inccrporate more than preclinical Behavioural Science, which is too easily forgotten or dismissed before practice begins. During the years of clinical training, input needs to be specifically integrated with the successive medical topics studied (Kelly, 1990). The current search in medical schools for vertical integration of subject matter across year levels assists continuing input during undergraduate years from psychologist academic/practitioners.

Workshops or other controlled rehearsal of communication skills are followed by taped interviews with simulated or real patients, with extensive but nonthreatening feedback (Thompson, 1984). Co-teaching by health psychologists and medical consultants demonstrates the cooperative and mutually respectful relationship between them. Information about local sources of specialist health psychologist expertise and how to access them can be given, issues of what behavioural techniques can be employed by doctors and which require psychological referral need exploration, and ideally discussions will occur when psychologists are not present, of case management plans with a clinical health psychology component. Research presentations can describe collaborative projects with psychologist and medical chief investigators. This variety of internship learning, via observation of and discussion with skilled practitioners and supervised practice, may present some problems for a while due to shortages of adequately experienced health psychologist practitioners.

Intercalated science degrees for medical students are becoming available in the larger educational centres, and offer the chance of more intensive instruction in health psychology. At postgraduate level too, health psychology should be available for study by medical graduates, based on their undergraduate Behavioural Science and associated studies, supplemented with extra study of research design and methodology, behaviour change techniques, and other pertinent topics. Graduates would be well-prepared for close collaboration with similarly intensively trained psychologists, preferably with overlapping courses.

System considerations

The length, content and teaching personnel in Behavioural Science courses vary widely according to the attitudes of senior consultants and more *ad hoc* determinants such as the availability of interested and capable teaching staff. Recognition of the need for patient-centred, humanistic medical practice has led to readiness to fit health psychology into curricula already acknowledged as over-burdened. However there are system-wide implications for one's view of the nature of medicine (discussed further below), which means that resistance to explicit health psychology content is likely from those with more traditional biomedical perspectives.

WHAT IMPACT WILL HEALTH PSYCHOLOGY TRAINING FOR MEDICAL STUDENTS HAVE?

Following their own recommendations, health psychologists in medical education will probably want to evaluate the impact of their efforts, in order to modify and improve them as required. It is at once apparent that several possible outcome measures exist. Some, such as student attendance at classes and conscientious preparation of assignments, seem to refer to the immediate impact of the teaching. They offer valuable feedback to the teacher about how the course is being received, how well its relevance to medical practice has been transmitted, and how much effort students have decided to invest in it. Such outcomes are analogous to patient/client satisfaction, or helping alliance measures from the early stages of psychotherapy: we know that these "immediate" outcomes are good predictors of longer-term ones. Certainly, health psychology teachers want to achieve more than student enthusiasm during the course – but unless this is achieved, other more distal outcomes become less likely.

As discussed above, the medical school as a system expresses its attitude to health psychology, and students will base their response to the course, partly on the indicators about its importance within medical training which are conveyed via the allocation of curriculum time, faculty resources, and the assessment arrangements.

Retention of knowledge past the examination, its incorporation into the students' cognitive framework, and the development of related skills, represent longer-term goals for health psychology teachers, the attainment of which is correspondingly harder to test. Performance criteria which are part of patient care can to some extent be specified. Examples are the student's ability to summarize the developmental challenges being faced by patients at certain ages, awareness of the role of stress and social isolation in the form and presentation of symptoms, ability to communicate clearly and supportively with patients, and mastery of behaviour change strategies suitable for routine use. Compliance and other "ultimate" goals such as lowered morbidity and mortality rates are affected by many other variables than the student's mastery of health psychology concepts, and are therefore not sufficiently specific outcome measures. Building followup assessment of health psychology teaching into the curriculum again implies a more than nominal level of commitment by the Faculty to its value.

Long-term effects of the permeation of medicine with health psychology

The development of health psychology has enormously expanded the field of application of psychological knowledge, and also offered unique opportunities for psychologists to expand the knowledge itself, for example by studying much more representative samples of people than previously. As a result, psychologists have realistically become more confident of being able to make valuable contributions to health care and the education of health care professionals.

Psychologists were first invited into medical schools to teach and treat in conjunction with psychiatrists. Clinical psychological assessment and therapy progressively expanded to include psychosomatic and other biopsychosocial disturbances. At the same time there was growing awareness within medical schools of the need to satisfy modern, better educated and more assertive patients by providing students with explicit education about doctor-patient communication, the effects of stress on health, attitude change, etc. Thus Behavioural Science courses were introduced, and more psychologists entered the medical school – at first mainly the familiar clinical psychologists then social psychologists, and even sociologists and anthropologists. Academic health psychologists then started to cooperate in research projects with the medical specialists around then, most of whom had had limited training in research methodology and statistical analysis. In a spiral process, the more psychologists did within the medical school, the greater their skills become and the more they were invited to do. Some credit for the development of health psychology must therefore go to the medical school establishment.

As psychologists became accepted within the medical schools, medical education itself was undergoing changes which mirrored different community expectations. Rigid divisions between preclinical and clinical subject matter began to disappear, explicit rather than casual observational training in interviewing or communication skills was accorded some then more curriculum time, and the status of primary care/family medicine slowly rose with the establishment of Departments, journals, and academic qualifications in general practice. Psychologists, independent of their initial sponsors the psychiatrists, now teach and research alongside representatives of every field of medical endeavour.

The potential gains for medicine of including health psychology within its training tend to be self-evident to psychologists. They relate to improvements in the effectiveness of patient care, and also to re-emphasis of its humanistic aspects, which drew many students to medicine in the first place and which has often been sorely missed by both students and practitioners (e.g. Conrad, 1988). The potential costs should not however be overlooked. Acceptance of a psychological view of the process of medical care complicates the simpler biomedical model and has far-reaching implications for subjects such as the doctor's status in relation to the patient and to psychologists, the place for microscopes versus mirrors in medical training, and public expectations of doctors.

Similarly, there are potential gains and losses for psychology of its expansion into medical education and research. Apart from the expanded subject pools and corresponding opportunities to develop and refine models of human behaviour, there is the chance to participate in a great humanitarian enterprise, namely the relief of suffering, on a wider scale than ever before. To be equal to this challenge, health psychology must work hard to grow in knowledge and skills, especially at the biological level and its integration into whole-person functioning, to expand its field of operations, and to restrain itself from unfounded or exaggerated claims.

The end result may therefore be considerable change in both medicine and health psychology – not in the form of a merger, but of mutual respect and acknowledgement of each other's specialist expertise, and a vigorous determination to keep abreast of relevant developments and apply them whenever appropriate.

SUMMARY

The basic undergraduate curriculum in medicine must contain enough information about health psychology for graduates to feel familiarity with its conceptual schemata, understand its clinical possibilities and how to tap into them via referral, and be able to incorporate appropriate techniques in their everyday practice. Starting with preclinical Behavioural Science type courses, and continuing through the clinical and postgraduate years of medical education, health psychology needs to be recognized as widely useful to medical practitioners, to have maximum impact. The results of growing mutual respect between medicine and health psychology are likely to bring substantial benefits to both disciplines.

References

Belar, C. D. (1990). Issues in training clinical health psychologists. *Psychology and Health*, **4**, 31–37.

Conrad, P. (1988). Learning to doctor: Reflections on recent accounts of the medical school years. *Journal of Health and Social Behavior*, *29*, 323–332.

Diekstra, R. F. W. (1990). Psychology, health and health care. *Psychology and Health*, **4**, 51–63.

Doherty, R. L. (1988). *Australian Medical Education and Workforce into the 21st Century.* Canberra: Australian Government Publishing Service.

Engel, G. L. (1982). The biopsychosocial model and medical education. Who are to be the teachers? *New England Journal of Medicine*, **306**, 802–805.

General Medical Council, Education Committee. (1987). *The Teaching of Behavioural Sciences, Community Medicine and General Practice in Basic Medical Education. Report of a Working Party.*

Kelly, M. P. (1990). A suitable case for *Technik*: Behavioural science in the postgraduate medical curriculum. *Medical Education*, **24**, 271–279.

Methorst, G. J., Jansen, M. A. and Kerkhof, J. F. M. (1990). Training in health psychology: An international look. *Psychology of Health*, **4**, 19–30.

Peay, M. Y. (1977). The use of clinical observations in the teaching of Behavioural Science. *Journal of Medical Education*, **52**, 685–686.

Stone, G. C. (1990). An international review of the emergence and development of health psychology. *Psychology and Health*, **4**, 3–17.

Taylor, S. E. (1990). Health psychology: The science and the field. *American Psychologist*, **45**, 40–50.

Thompson, J. (1984). Communicating with patients. In R. Fitzpatrick, J. Hinton, S. Newman, G.

Scambler, and J. Thompson (eds.), *The Experience of Illness*, London: Tavistock, pp. 87–108.
Weinman, J. (1989). A survey of pre-clinical psychology teaching in United Kingdom medical schools. *Medical Education*, **23**, 77–80.
Winefield, H. R. (1981). Behavioural Science in the medical curriculum: Why and how. In M. J. Christie and P. G. Mellett (eds.), *Foundations of Psychosomatics*, London: Wiley, pp. 15–38.
Winefield, H. R. (1990). The Child Study: A multipurpose practical project in Behavioural Science. *Medical Teacher* **12,** 95–97.

CHAPTER 13

IMPLEMENTING A BEHAVIORAL MEDICINE PROGRAM IN AN INTERNAL MEDICINE RESIDENCY: A DESCRIPTION OF CURRICULUM CONTENT, RESOURCES AND BARRIERS ENCOUNTERED

JOHN CHRISTENSEN

Behavioral Medicine Training Coordinator, Internal Medicine Residency Program Good Samaritan Hospital and Medical Center, 1015 N.W. 22nd Avenue, Portland, Oregon 97210

WENDY LEVINSON

Associate Director Internal Medicine Training Program, Assistant Professor Oregon Health Sciences University, Good Samaritan Hospital and Medical Center, 1015 N.W. 22nd Avenue, Portland, Oregon 97210

Many internal medicine training programs are currently developing curricula designed to teach the psychosocial aspects of patient care and doctor-patient communication skills. However, faculty may lack expertise regarding how to accomplish new educational goals in these areas. This article is designed to assist programs by describing in detail how a comprehensive behavioral medicine program was integrated into a general internal medicine program at a university-affiliated community hospital. It describes the program goals, resources needed, content included, obstacles to implementation and potential solutions to the problems encountered.

There is increasing concern in internal medicine training programs about how to develop curricula focusing on the psychosocial aspects of patient care and doctor-patient communication skills. The American Boarc of Internal Medicine has recently mandated programs to certify the humanistic skills of trainees (American Board of Internal Medicine, 1985). But how should training directors develop appropriate curricula? Traditional training programs may find themselves ill-equipped in terms of faculty or knowledge about how to design a comprehensive curriculum integrated with their existing program.

The goal of this article is to describe how a behavioral medicine program was integrated into a general internal medicine program at Good Samaritan Hospital and Medical Center (GSH and MC), a university-affiliated community hospital in Portland, Oregon. The program includes 28 residents in the three years of training. The article is designed to provide a description of the program goals, resources needed, content included, obstacles to implementation and approaches to problems encountered.

PROGRAM GOALS

The goals of the behavioral medicine curriculum, initiated in October, 1984, are as follows:

1) Fostering in the training program a holistic, patient centered perspective that includes consideration of the biological, psychological and social contexts of illness and wellness.
2) Increasing physician-patient communication skills.
3) Instilling in the medical faculty an awareness of the key role of communication skills in the practice of medicine and the methodology to teach these skills to residents during clinical supervision.
4) Increasing skills in identifying and managing psychiatric disorders in the context of primary care.
5) Increasing residents' fund of knowledge about the behavioral aspects of illness and medical treatment.
6) Enhancing residents' attention to their own mental health and their skills at managing stress.

HISTORY OF THE BEHAVIORAL MEDICINE PROGRAM

The behavioal medicine program has evolved over the course of six years. Beginning in 1981 there emerged a recognition of the need for augmented resident education in behavioral medicine. This need was addressed by the addition of weekly behavioral medicine rounds, occasional noon conferences and informal evening sessions devoted to psychological difficulties of resident training. Although these teaching sessions were helpful in increasing resident sensitivity to behavioral issues, the faculty agreed that a more formal behavioral medicine curriculum should be incorporated into the training program. With the award of a Public Health Service General Internal Medicine training grant in 1984, a behavioral medicine team was added to the faculty. This team included a clinical psychologist coordinator and a psychiatric nurse practitioner. A psychiatrist served as a consultant to the program. It is with the guidance of these people that the curriculum described in this article has been developed.

FACILITIES AND EQUIPMENT

The outpatient clinics are the primary settings for training in behavioral medicine. One clinic is located in the hospital, and the other is a neighborhood satellite clinic in a medically underserved area of Portland. Residents spend 25% of their training in these clinics seeing patients for whom they provide ongoing longitudinal care. Both clinics are equipped with a videotape camera, monitor and one-way mirror.

CURRICULUM CONTENT AND IMPLEMENTATION STRATEGIES

Communication and interviewing skills training

The important of teaching communication skills in a medical curriculum has been well-established (DiMatteo, M. R., 1979; Carroll, J. G. and Monroe, J., 1980; Waitzkin, H., 1984; Lipkin, M., Jr., Quill, T. and Napodano, R. J., 1984). Formal training and supervision in communication and interviewing skills is a central component of our behavioral medicine curriculum. Key skills that have been targeted are listed in Table 1. Interviewing skills are taught primarily during clinical supervision of residents in the outpatient clinics, where residents are observed interviewing patients. Frequently, interviews are videotaped and later reviewed with the resident.

Table 1 Interviewing and communication skills.

1) Forming hypotheses about patient's beliefs concerning symptoms and illness.
   A) Locus of control
   B) Reification vs. process
   C) Expectations for change
   D) Ecology of illness (psychosocial context)

2) Nonverbal behavior
   A) Decoding of patient's internal states (e.g., gestures, facial expression, voice tone, breathing pattern)
   B) Encoding of physician's affect with accuracy (e.g., gestures, facial expression, voice tone)
   C) Rapport-building behaviors (e.g., matching voice volume and tempo, timing of gestures, breathing in unison)

3) Linguistic skills
   A) Open-ended vs. closed questions
   B) Indirect suggestion
   C) Active listening (summarizing, reflecting feelings, echoing patient's phrases)
   D) Reframing
   E) Individualizing amount and level of information given
   F) Timing of physician utterances (e.g., pauses, interruptions)

4) Awareness of transference and countertransference
   A) Understanding the patient's affect as information
   B) Increased awareness of physician's own affective states and value systems as related to patient states

Videotape review is a valuable educational tool as it allows direct review of aspects of the interview that are not accessible to the observer's recall. For example, correlation of nonverbal postural changes and shifts in facial expression between psysician and patient can be detected when the videotape is replayed in fast speed, thus allowing observation of the degree of rapport established in the interview. Furthermore, residents may observe their own medical interviewing technique and stop the tape at various choice points to experiment with differernt approaches. Videotape provides a focus both on the process as well as content of the interview.

New interns are introduced to the medical interviewing curriculum during their initial orientation to the hospital. A three-hour conference on their first day includes a demonstration of the use of role playing techniques by faculty and small group work utilizing role play to learn a sample of communication skills. This session also allows interns to introduce themselves and to discuss their feelings about beginning the program.

To further emphasize the importance of medical interviewing skills and to concentrate the training in this area, an annual full-day retreat is held, early in the academic year, at a location away from the hospital. Physicians are hired to provide hospital coverage, so that the residents on-call can attend. A more extensive descrition of this retreat can be found in another article (Christensen, J. F., Levinson, W., Colligan, J. L., Dunn, P. M., Jones, S. R. and Morgenstern, A., 1987). Material covered includes expression of empathy in difficult circumstances, attending to one's own internal distractions, communication influences on medical decision-making, persuading patients to undergo difficult procedures, and the use of videotaped feedback in clinical supervision.

We have found the residents receptive to learning communication skills while working with their own clinic patients. Particularly when they feel at an impasse with a difficult patient, residents are eager to try alternative approaches. Frequently residents will videotape their work with such patients, and later review the tape with a supervisor to learn new communication strategies. The commitment to teaching medical interviewing in the clinic setting has been an important factor in increasing resident interest. In addition, as will be discussed below, the internists supervising in the clinic integrate discussion of communication skills with their attention to diagnostic and management issues. This integration also contributes to resident interest in learning these skills.

Training of medical faculty in methods of teaching interviewing skills

Many opportunities for teaching residents to improve communication skills occur during clinical supervison by the medical faculty. Since these communication skills are veiwed in our training program as integral to the art of medical practice, it is important that they not be relegated to a separate discipline and separate teaching segment under the rubric of "behavioral medicine." Hence, it is critical that the medical faculty be both sensitive to and trained in the techniques of teaching effective doctor-patient communication skills.

For this purpose the clinical psychologist provides supervision in communication techniques to faculty members as requested. He meets weekly with the Associate Program Director to review videotapes of patient interactions and to increase her skills at teaching medical interviewing. In addition, in January of 1986, of three-day intensive workshop on teaching medical interviewing was sponsored by the Department of Medicine for all faculty responsible for residency training in Portland. This workshop was presented by the Society for General Internal Medicine (SGIM), Task Force for the Medical Interview. The result of this workshop was increased interest and enthusiasm for teaching communication skills on the part of the medical faculty at GSH and MC and the establishment of a monthly meeting of faculty from all the residency training programs in the city. These meetings include time for sharing teaching techniques, as well as time for the faculty to critique each other's interviewing skills. In June, 1987, the National Faculty Development Course on Teaching Medical Interviewing (Sponsored by SGIM) was held as GSH and MC. The participation of six of our faculty in this course further developed faculty skills, cohesion, and commitment to this teaching in our program.

Additionally, the medical faculty has received training in the fundamentals of Neurolinguistic Programming (NLP) from a nationally recognized trainer in this methodology. NLP is a method of observing, assessing and utilizing an individual's unique style of learning and communicating. (Christensen, J.F., Levinson, W. and Grinder, M., 1990) As applied to medical interviewing, it provides the physician with strategies for maximizing rapport and patient compliance. Following their training, the faculty have incorporated some of this methodology into their clinic supervison.

Managing psychological disorders in medical settings

Many patients seeking care from a physician have an emotional or psychological disorder that is either a primary problem or ancillary to their medical problems (Regier, D. A., Goldberg, I. D. and Taube, C. A., 1987; Hoeper, E. W., Nycz, G. R., Cleary, P. D., Regier, D. A. and Goldberg, I. D., 1979; Thompson, T. L., Stoudemire, A., Mitchell, W. D. and Grant, R. L., 1983). Our goal is to teach residents to recognize the types of psychological disorder most likely to be seen in medical practice. It is important that they be able to identify a psychological problem, provide brief intervention through counseling or pharmacotherapy, manage bahvioral problems that occur during medical care, and refer patients for professional mental health treatment when that is warranted.

Teaching in this area occurs formally during monthly behavioral medicine noon conferences and informally during clinical supervision of residents in the outpatient clinic and on the hospital wards. Over the course of three years an attempt is made to cover a broad spectrum of relevant clinic topics. A representative sample of noon conference topics is listed in Table 2.

Table 2 Behavioral medicine noon conferences.

Alcoholism and substance abuse†
Depression†
Managing the suicidal patient†
Mental status exam†
Overview of DSM–III and taking a psychological history†
Anxiety disorders
Drug seeking behavior in addicts
Factitious disorders
Eating disorders
Managing the hostile/violent patient
Manic-depressive illness
Personality disorders
Psychogenic illnesses/somatoform disorders
Referrals for mental health treatment
Sexual problems

† Topics covered early in the year the interns.

In our experience the most significant learning about management of psychological disorders occurs during supervision of residents on individual cases in the outpatient clinic. For example, in that setting a resident can follow a depressed patient over time and witness the changes that occur with appropriate behavioral and pharmacological interventions. The clinical psychologist or mental health nurse practitioner sometimes model to the resident how to work with a particular problem. With more experienced residents, faculty may observe or videotape the interview through the one-way mirror and later give feedback to the resident. Often the resident is given an article pertinent to a particular patient's psychological disorder. In addition, at a weekly conference residents informally present patients they have seen in the clinic to their peers and faculty. These conferences allow opportunities for the behavioral medicine faculty to teach the group by focusing on individual patient care problems.

Personality and behavioral correlates of specific illnesses

Many illnesses encountered in medical practice are intertwined with personality and behavioral factors. These factors may be either precursors influencing the individual's susceptibility to an organic disorder or emotional consequences of the medical condition. In didactic sessions (Table 3) and during case supervision, residents are taught to recognize behavioral patterns that predispose to physical illness. For example, at a conference on the Type A coronary-prone behavior pattern residents first completed the Jenkins Activity Survey and Framingham Scale to assess the extent of their own Type-A pattern. This created high interest that facilitated learning about this pattern, since they were naturally curious about what pertained to their own manner of coping. Familiarity with this information can help residents begin to think about preventive measures they can implement with their ongoing patients, such as relaxation training for chronic anxiety and other forms of stress management.

Table 3 Didactic sessions on personality and behavioral aspects of illness.

A) Precursors of illness
Behavioral immunology
Type A coronary-prone behavior pattern
B) Consequences of illness
Emotional problems associated with AIDS
Behavioral oncology
Behavioral management of chronic pain
Low back pain
Strategies for working with the dying patient and family†
C) Patient management
Maximizing patient compliance
Uses of hypnosis in medicine

† Topic covered early in the year for interms.

Residents are also instructed on the emotional sequelae of chronic illnesses. For example, many residents are treating AIDS patients, who must cope with anxiety, depression and a radical change in self-concept. Early in the year a noon conference is devoted to the issue of working with dying patients and the grief of their families. The behavioral medicine faculty work with residents individually as they deal with particular dying patients.

Special attention is focused on the issue of patient compliance. Part of the instruction in the area of communication skills involves ways of negotiating a treatment contract with the patient. This information has taken place both in a didactic session and as a component of the previously mentioned communication skills retreat. Nonverbal techniques designed to increase compliance are taught routinely in the course of clinical supervision in the clinics. Specific compliance problems that necessitate a complex array of interventions, such as smoking cessation, are discussed as special topics in a conference.

Resident mental health

The rigors of a residency in internal medicine present several stressors that tax the coping resources of house officers and increase their vulnerability to emotional distress (Clark, D. C., Salazar-Grueso, E., Grabler, P. and Fawcett, J., 1984; Valko, R. J. and Clayton, P. J., 1975; Alexander, D., Monk, J. S. and Jonas, A. P., 1985). In recognition of the impact of these predictable stressors on residents' emotions, several activities have been initiated to increase the personal and program resources available to house staff. Periodic retreats were initiated in the Summer of 1985 to address the issue of resident mental health. These retreats, which are a half-day in length, are held three times a year on a regular work day. A physician is hired to manage hospital responsibilities so all the house officers can attend. These retreats are conducted away from the hospital, either at a retreat center or a relaxed home setting. The format has involved a keynote address followed by small group discussions on topics related to stressors and ways of coping. Some of the topics address the transition experienced by new interns, the challenges of second year residents assuming a new role of supervision and teaching, and conflict between one's professional role and personal life. A valuable function of these small group discussions is to legitimize the awareness of the stressors inherent in residency and to provide a basis for ongoing support between colleagues. The day also involves time for physical recreation and socializing, which residents have valued highly given the minimal time ordinarily available for these activities.

Throughout the year the behavioral medicine faculty facilitate a monthly group meeting of the interns, which allows time for ventilation of frustrations, problem-solving of commonly shared issues and teaching individual coping strategies such as self-hypnosis and relaxation skills. These meetings are kept confidential, and an attempt is made to establish a secure, non-threatening environment in which problems can be addressed. A problem with these sessions is that they require a shift of the intern's attention and energy level from the intense time pressures of managing patient care to the focus on their own emotions and needs. This is particularly problematic when the session is held in the middle of a work day. Nevertheless, several residents have indicated that they value this time together, and last year's intern group elected to continue these monthly group meetings as second-year residents. For this group the focus shifted to the stress involved in becoming teachers and supervisors of interns, and their monthly meetings involve case discussions of difficulties encountered in their teaching responsibilities.

Individual counseling of residents is also provided by the behavioral medicine faculty. This counseling is maintained confidential by department policy. Individual sessions may originate by request of a resident or by the faculty if a particular resident appears to be having emotional or interpersonal problems. If the resident requires extended psychotherapy, he or she is referred to a private therapist.

BARRIERS TO IMPLEMENTING BEHAVIORAL MEDICINE TRAINING

Any innovation tends to encounter natural resistance. With time, the habituation of resident and faculty to "the way things are done here" allows unconscious, automatic programs for behavior to take over as the mores of the system are learned. Adding a new training component initially required more time and conscious thought to incorporate new patterns of interacting with patients, a new and unfamiliar language, and a different approach to learning and teaching.

Initial attitudes of residents toward the introduction of behavioral medicine were a mixture of openness, skepticism and opposition. Those who opposed it tended to perceive behavioral skills as not traditionally a part of medicine, regarded it as "soft" vs. "hard" science, and tended to be threatened by a focus on their communication skills. Some expressed the attitude that they already had good "people skills" before going into medicine. A key to overcoming this resistance was individual supervision of residents in the clinic, where behavioral skills helped to resolve issues with problem patients. Success with difficult patients led residents to view the assistance of the behavioral medicine faculty as relevant to their patient care. Care was taken to provide supervision on doctor-patient communication in a non-threatening way, pointing out positive skills and reinforcing the notion that there are choice points in an interview with multiple correct ways to proceed.

A particularly difficult barrier to full acceptance of behavioral medicine was the resistance or indifference of a few key residents who were perceived by their peers and faculty as being role models. These residents had influence over the attitudes of many of their peers, and winning them over presented a challenge. The most vocal critics were invited to form a bahavioral medicine advisory committee, designed to provide suggestions for curriculum development. In general the philosophy of the behavioral medicine program has been to involve residents in planning conferences and retreats. As the "critics" have assumed more planning responsibility with the guidance of the faculty, they have manifested a sense of ownership over the behavioral training component.

Attitudes of internal medicine faculty were also a significant barrier to implementation of the behavioral medicine training. Unless behavioral skills are reinforced throughtout the learning environment, residents do not attend as carefully to their acquisition. With involvement of the internal medicine faculty, psychological skills become woven into the fabric of medical training. Increasing medical faculty involvement in teaching interviewing skills has been a key to a positive shift in resident attitudes toward behavioral medicine. Factors that led to this increased role for some of the core medical faculty were their participation in the medical interviewing course, the faculty training in NLP, individual supervision and review of videotapes of faculty interviews by the psychologist, participation in behavioral medicine conferences, and the support of the chief of medicine.

Another barrier is the perception by both residents and medical faculty that behavioral issues and communication skills take too much time. The initial investment of time required in learning a new skill was made more palatable for the residents doing clinic rotations by setting aside weekly supervision hours in their clinic schedule. The residents come to view this as a time in which they can be free of patient care and devote more relaxed attention to this learning. As residents become familiar with behavioral skills, they discover that it actually saves them time in patient interviews and that they can create a climate of empathy in which the patients perceive they have been given a lot of time when the actual clock time is shorter.

Residents initially were resistant to having their patient interactions videotaped for a variety of reasons. Before the addition of a one-way mirror into the clinic, the video camera was set up in an examination room. The presence of the camera was both intrusive and took up space, requiring resident and patient to sit close together in an unnaturally constrained manner. The one-way mirror took the camera out of the exam room, alleviating this problem. Another barrier was the need to get the patient's written consent. Residents felt that asking patients for their consent interfered with their rapport. Currently the nurses obtain the patient's consent and set up the video system, thus freeing the resident of these constraints. In addition, resident perceptions of videotaping as an evaluative tool increased their apprehension. This perception was altered over time by having faculty members tape their interviews for review in conferences. Care is taken that videotape review is done with a sense of curiosity and learning, that choice points in the interview are discussed with a sense of options rather than right or wrong responses, and that evaluative comments are kept to a minimum. Furthermore, residents gradually have been desensitized to the video equipment by using it in multiple settings, such as taping interesting ward cases for presentation at morning report, taping family members during house staff functions, and preparing skits for the year-end party.

A significant early barrier was the difficulty of integrating non-medical faculty, the psychologist and nurse practitioner, into the teaching program. This difficulty stemmed from attitudes of the house staff, the medical faculty, and the non-medical behavioral medicine faculty. Attitudes of residents shifted favorably over time because of the relevance of the behavioral medicine supervision to patient care and because of the role of the non-medical faculty in organizing house staff retreats and providing individual counseling. As the medical faculty became more involved in the learning and teaching of behavioral medicine, their acceptance of the non-medical faculty increased. Although initially the non-medical faculty felt like "strangers in a strange land" in the predominantly medical environment, they recognized with time the unique contributions they could make. As house staff began initiating more supervision requests and as the new faculty became more familiar with the medical training environment, the initial feelings of distance were bridged.

Finally, there were barriers to implementing a program for resident mental health. There is a natural resistance that young and perfectionistic residents have to revealing their own sense of frustration and inadequacy. The tendency is to perceive one's peers as more competent and to perceive disclosure of emotional distress as a sign of weakness. The house staff retreats and the monthly stress management groups, with their emphasis on legitimizing the predictable stressors and emotional distress of residency, have helped open residents to the values of self-disclosure. In addition, the establishment of a clear department policy of confidentiality in the individual counseling of residents dissolved their concerns that the behavioral faculty were agents of the department of medicine and would report back to the faculty problems disclosed in counseling sessions.

RESIDENT EVALUATION

Systematic evaluation of resident competence and progress in communication skills has been problematic. Although various scales for rating of clinical interviews have been developed (Carroll, J. G. and Monroe, J., 1980; Robbins, A. S., Kauss, D. R., Heinrich, R., Abrass, I., Dreyer, J. and Clyman, B., 1979; National Board of Medical Examiners, 1981), they are time consuming for faculty. Clinical ratings by attending physicians are performed at the end of each rotation, using the standard rating forms of the American Board of Internal Medicine. The item referring to Attitude and Interpersonal Skills, however, is nonspecific and of doubtful reliability. Currently, there is a lack of simple quantitative evaluation tools to measure house staff competence in communication skills. Given these limitations, the present evaluation of residents' progress is subjective and non-quantitative. The evaluation of residents' progress occurs primarily in their supervision with the behavioral medicine faculty at regular intervals over the three years.

An educational activity that may provide a basis for future resident evaluation is the practice of giving residents their own videotapes on which to record patient interviews sequentially. These individual tapes allow the progress of each resident's interviewing skills to be observed over time. An application of a standardized interview rating scale to these serial interviews may offer a measure of resident progress. In addition, a standardized patient program (Stillman, P. L., Swanson, D. B., Smee, S., Stillman, A. E., Ebert, T. H., Emmel, V. S., Caslowitz, J., Greene, H. L., Hamolsky, M., Hatem, C., Levenson, D. J., Levin, R., Levinson, G., Ley, B., Morgan, G. J., Parrino, T., Robinson, S. and Willms, J., 1986) has been developed and this has been provided has another form of objective evaluation.

FUTURE DIRECTIONS

Future development of the behavioral medicine training program is anticipated in faculty development, resident selection, resident evaluation, long-range funding and cooperation among local training programs.

To further educate the medical faculty in the fundamentals of behavioral science, a weekly seminar has recently been instituted for interested faculty. This seminar is an informal discussion of readings selected by the behavioral medicine faculty, covering broad areas such as the history of psychology and the major theoretical approaches to psychopathology and psychotherapy, as well as specific applications of behavioral theory to medicine. This will be an ongoing seminar responding to the interests and inclinations of the faculty.

Attempts will be made to attract residents to the program with a special interest in behavioral medicine. A core group of such residents may constitute a catalyst for further extending the scope of behavioral training.

A future challenge will be developing funding sources after the Public Health Service funding ends. Hospital administrators are often reluctant to devote more resources than present allocations to resident education. Hence, it will be important to establish other sources including local charitable agencies, fund raising through benefit auctions, and marketing of educational services to the medical community.

CONCLUSION

In the last few decades mastery of the technological innovations in medicine has often overshadowed the human dimension. Competence in medicine demands of the physician an equivalent mastery of the psychological and social contexts of illness and wellness. It demands attention to the art as well as the science of healing.

The art of healing is not an elusive construct, but a definable domain with specific areas of content and process skills. It is the experience of the residency training program at GSH and MC that this domain can be integrated into a general internal medicine residency and that the skills are teachable. The core of this integration has occurred in the outpatient setting and has utilized the residents' experience with their own patients. The implementation of this program has encountered certain barriers eventually surmounted by strategies that may be generalizable to other teaching programs.

The learning of psychosocial skills is not simply a matter of digesting information or of observing and practicing a set of techniques. The pivotal moment of this learning is an act of self-discovery, in which the resident becomes aware of resources within his or her history that have a healing impact on the present encounter with the patient. After all the teaching, videotaping, role playing, supervision and reading, there is a sense of contact in which the uniqueness of the physician interacts with the uniqueness of the patient in a manner that promotes health and growth. The teaching faculty can provide the conditions and lead the resident to this wellspring, but the assimilation remains a highly personal experience.

Recently a resident related an incident of such a discovery. Toward the end of a busy day in the clinic she was asked to see a patient who was in distress because of abdominal pain and who had a history of taxing the coping resources of the staff by her histrionic style. the resident's impulse was to expedite the interview by ignoring the patient's complaining and giving her a pain medication. The resident, however, decided to experiment with newly learned communication skills. She found that she was able to shift the patient from a highly emotional, complaining mode to a cooperative one. This allowed the resident eventually to arrive at a diagnosis of an organic basis for the patient's pain and plan a successful treatment. The transaction ended with satisfaction for both resident and patient. In telling the story the resident was obviously pleased with her own skill at establishing rapport with a difficult patient at a point when the resident's energy was at a low ebb. Her expectations of the outcome of similar future situations had significantly changed. Episodes such as this one have helped support the teaching faculty in our conviction that behavioral skills can be taught to residents and incorporated into their daily practice.

References

Alexander, D., Monks, J. S. and Jonas, A. P. (1985) Occupational stress, personal strain, and coping among residents and faculty members. *Journal of Medical Education,* **60,** 830–839.

American Board of Internal Medicine (1985) *A guide to awareness and evaluation of humanistic qualities in the internist.* Portland, OR

Carroll, J. G. and Monroe, J. (1980) Teaching clinical interviewing in the health professions: a review of empirical research. *Evaluation of Health Professionals,* **3**(1), 2145

Christensen, J. F., Levinson, W., Colligan, J. L., Dunn, P. M., Jones, S. R. and Morgenstern, A. (1987) A one-day communication workshop for internal medicine residents. *Journal of Medical Education,* **62,** 687–690

Christensen, J.F., Levinson, W. and Grinder, M. (1990) Applications of Neurolinguistic Programming to medicine. *Journal of General Internal Medicine,* **5,** 522–527.

Clark, D. C., Salazar-Grueso, E., Grabler, P. and Fawcett, J. (1984) Predictors of depression during the first six months of internship. *American Journal of Psychiatry,* **141**(9), 1095–1098

Di Matteo, M. R. (1979) A social-psychological analysis of physician-patient rapport: Toward a science of the art of medicine. *Journal of Social Issues,* **35**(1), 12–33

Hoeper, E. W., Nycz, G. R., Cleary, P. D., Regier, D. A. and Goldberg, I. D. (1979) Estimated prevalence of RDC mental disorder in primary medical care. *International Journal of Mental Health,* **8,** 6–15

Lipkin, M., Jr., Quill, T. and Napodano, R. J. (1984) The medical interview: a core curriculum for residencies in internal medicine. *Annals of Internal Medicine,* **100,** 277–284

National Board of Medical Examiners (1981) *Interaction System for Interview Evaluation,* Philadelphia, PA

Regier, D. A., Goldberg, I. D. and Taube, C. A. (1987) De facto U.S. mental health services system. *Archives of General Psychiatry,* **35,** 685–693

Robbins, A. S., Kauss, D. R., Heinrich, R., Abrass, I., Dreyer, J. and Clyman, B. (1979) Interpersonal skills training: evaluation in an internal medicine residency. *Journal of Medical Education,* **54,** 885–894

Stillman, P. L., Swanson, D. B., Smee, S., Stillman, A. E., Ebert, T. H., Emmel, V. S., Caslowitz, J., Greene, H. L., Hamolsky, M., Hatem, C., Levenson, D. J., Levin, R., Levinson, G., Ley, B., Morgan, G. J., Parrino, T., Robinson, S. and Willms, J. (1986) Assessing clinical skills with standardized patients. *Annals of Internal Medicine,* **105,** 762–771

Thompson, T. L., Stoudemire, A., Mitchell, W. D. and Grant, R. L. (1983) Underrecognition of patient's psychosocial distress in a university hospital medical clinic. *American Journal of Psychiatry,* **140,** 158–161

Valko, R. J. and Clayton, P. J. (1975) Depression in the internship. *Diseases of the Nervous System,* **36,** 26–29

Waitzkin, H. (1984) Doctor-patient communication: clinical implications of social scientific research. *The Journal of American Medical Association,* **252,** 2441–2446

SECTION FOUR

CONCLUDING OVERVIEWS

CHAPTER 14

DETERMINANTS OF HEALTH PSYCHOLOGY'S DEVELOPMENT

JOHN WEINMAN

Unit of Psychology, United Medical and Dental Schools of Guy's and St Thomas' Hospitals, University of London, London Bridge, London SE1 9RT

This paper attempts to predict key developments in health psychology over the next few years. It does so by considering some of the important forces which are likely to determine the nature of progress in theory and practice. Thus it is anticipated that, in addition to progress within the discipline, health psychology will develop in response to a range of societal changes and needs as well as to priorities and progress within medicine. A key issue will involve the planning and implementation of effective training in order to establish core undergraduate and postgraduate curricula, with the latter resulting in the professional arrival of health psychology.

Forecasting the future of any discipline is a difficult task. With a field as new and fast-growing as health psychology, it is particularly problematic. This chapter attempts this task by focusing on some of the determinants of future developments in health psychology, as a basis for considering the sorts of changes which are both likely and desirable. The shape of health psychology in the next decade will be influenced and determined by many forces including the needs of society and developments within medicine as well as by pressures within discipline. A selection of these influences and determinants is presented to provide a picture of the range of issues involved.

SOCIETAL DETERMINANTS OF FUTURE DEVELOPMENTS

A general societal determinant as regards health arises from the challenging statement of the Alma Ata Declaration of the World Health Organisation (WHO), which aimed at providing health for all by the year 2000 (WHO, 1981). Although this raises all sorts of questions as to what is meant by health, the WHO were postulating a level of health which permitted a socially and productive life. In an earlier chapter Diekstra notes that achieving this very laudable aim will necessitate a major emphasis on psychosocial and behavioural approaches to health maintenance and health care, using the primary care setting as the main context

As a basic step in meeting the WHO challenge, health psychologists will need to continue producing good research indentifying the health risks associated with different behaviours and social conditions. This data should then be used in attempts to lobby politicians and other policy makers since it is clear that political, economic and social changes will have to occur in attempting to eliminate conditions such as poverty, unemployment and loneliness, all potent sources of ill health. Since many high risk individual behaviours (e.g. smoking; poor diet; high alcohol consumption) are often associated with these adverse social conditions, it will be quite inappropriate for health psychologists to pursue individual models of behaviour change as the only way of achieving 'health for all'. It will be necessary to adopt community-based approaches and to develop a better understanding of the social meanings of different risk behaviours and of the norms and value systems which underpin and maintain them. It will also be necessary to act to put pressure on such different groups and organisations as local politicians, food distributors, the media and environmental policy makers in order to provide a social climate in which it becomes easier for the individual to make health-related choices and to achieve health-related behaviour change (e.g. Elder, Abrams, Beaudin et al, 1988).

In order to grasp this particular nettle, health psychologists will need to have a clear understanding of such fields as epidemiology and consumer behaviour, as well as of the ways of which social conditions impinge on health and health-related behaviour. This obviously has implications for training in health psychology which is discussed below.

Another major societal need arises from the changing demographic structure of industrialised societies during this century and the very significant increase in the proportion of elderly people. It is clear that health psychologists must devote a clear research priority to the investigation of health cognitions, health behaviour and health needs in older people (e.g. Amir, 1987). It will also be necessary to understand more about the influence of social contexts, to develop greater insights into the problems experienced by the carers of elderly people and to develop effective interventions. Moreover, to obviate the various problems associated with cross-sectional studies, it will be held vital to initiate longitudinal studies of behaviour and health. In this way it will be possible to become more confident that our prescriptions for such healthy life-style changes as regular exercise actually do result in positive health outcomes in old age (e.g. Howard, 1989).

Another very differrent social trend has been the increased awareness of environmental or 'green' issues, which have radical implications for our future health. Here the major changes will clearly have to come from governments and industrial companies but we should not underestimate the power of effective lobbying. Health psychologists can contribute by producing research demonstrating effects of adverse environmental conditions and toxins on health and behaviour. Moreover, there is a very practical role to be played in increasing public awareness of the extent to which behaviour change can produce positive environmental outcomes. For example, demonstrable benefits will occur if people can be persuaded to change transport habits from private to public transport, to use fuels and power sources which are environmentally less hazardous and to save such materials as glass and paper for re-cycling.

A very notable feature of the political landscape in many countries has been the emergence of effective 'green' lobbies and political parties. It is hoped that health psychologists will be able to contribute to this process by offering knowledge, skills and support to the many policies these groups are pursuing since they do provide an important route to the maintenance of health and the prevention of future health hazards.

DEVELOPMENTS IN MEDICINE

Here again a brief selection of trends and issues will serve to provide different examples of some future directions for the development of health psychology. Thus this section will focus on important health problems, emergent medical technologies and on better ways of evaluating patients' quality of life and responses to treatment.

It is very likely that the most salient health problem in terms of medical research and public interest will continue to be in the area of Human Immunodeficiency Virus (HIV) and the Acquired Immune Deficiency Syndrome (AIDS). Psychologists should be able to make a contribution to two distinct aspects of HIV/AIDS. The first is in the area of primary prevention, particularly since this is currently the major option for limiting the spread of the disease. Attempts to do this have involved a range of mass media campaigns which have achieved some change in the knowledge of sexually active young people but generally there has been little significant behaviour change directly resulting from such campaigns (e.g. Sherr, 1987; Rigby et al, 1989). Thus there is a major challenge for health psychologists to become involved in the planning of effective preventive campaigns. A second challenge is to understand the role of behavioural factors in the progression of HIV/AIDS. There have been some studies of the effects of life events on people with AIDS and there is growing evidence of the potential contribution of such factors as relaxation, dietary change and coping. Here good, longitudinal studies are needed to evaluate the extent to which psychological variables can affect both emotional and biological outcomes. These, in turn, can provide the basis for developing effective psychological interventions for improving coping and, hopefully, delaying the progression of the disease. It also may provide valuable insights for the growing field of psychoneuroimmunology but, as Temoshok (1990) notes there are considerable methodological and other difficulties in using AIDS as a framework or a model for studying psychological influences on the immune system.

An undoubted second major development in medicine, with implications for health psychology, is in the practical application of the so-called 'new genetics', and the use of genetic probes either to identify individuals who are 'at risk' of developing major diseases or for prenatal diagnosis. There are many considerations here, which have been discussed in detail elsewhere (Weinman, in press). The task for health psychologists will be to investigate the various psychological issues associated with this type of screening and to understand more clearly how individuals make sure of and cope with the information which is revealed. This will be needed to facilitate the difficult decision-making tasks involved (e.g. whether to plan a family; to terminate a pregnancy, etc.) and to provide good counselling approaches which are appropriate for dealing with these complex questions.

Another major technical advance in medicine which offers scope for challenging psychological research is in the area of medical computing. Computers are being used increasingly for the storage of medical records, automating laboratory analyses and for interviewing patients and providing diagnostic information. It is the latter task which is of most interest and concern to psychologists and should draw upon the expertise of cognitive and health psychologists. Cognitive scientists are already engaged in the task of studying and defining medical expertise so that this expertise can be transformed into viable computer programs (e.g. Hunter, 1984). Health psychologists will need to provide insights about the different functions of the medical consultation and to investigate the effects of human computer interaction on patients and staff. It will be necessary to know whether an interrogation by computer gives rise to qualitatively and quantitatively different data and to find out how the decisions made by computers are evaluated by patients as well as the extent to which they are implemented and acted upon.

The final area in medicine which psychologists will need to make a key contribution is in the evaluation of 'quality of life'. Increasingly the development of new treatments calls into question their effects on the patients' quality of life. It is no longer sufficient for clinicians to state that a treatment is successful in terms of its effects on a specific biological process (e.g. tumour growth; cardiac functioning, etc) but it is also vital to know whether it gives rise to a significant improvement in the way in which someone lives. This growing realisation should open the door for some important psychological research to identify the important components of life quality, as well as the need to develop valid new measures for assessing this (see Fallowfield, 1990). This is an area where good models are required and where psychologists need to make use of the insights from work on patients' illness and health cognitions (e.g. Leventhal, Meyer and Nerenz, 1980) in order to develop assessments which take account of individual perceptions and priorities.

DEVELOPMENTS WITHIN HEALTH PSYCHOLOGY

In terms of its disciplinary development, it will be important for health psychology to generate and make use of coherent models of health and behaviour (Marteau and Johnston, 1987). In particular, a basic requirement is the need to construct core models of health cognitions as a basis for understanding health behaviours. There is also a real need for health psychologists to begin to reach some consensus as to the nature and measurement of the core concepts in the discipline. Concepts such as coping, social support and life stress are used and assessed very differently across studies which means that it is often difficult to compare or combine findings. Although it is necessary to try out and dvelop new ways of conceptualising and measuring important processes it is also worthwhile for time and effort to be spent carrying out good meta-analyses and critical reviews (e.g. Cohen, 1987; Schwarzer and Leppin, 1989). Hopefully the result of this will be a greater awareness of the strengths and weaknesses of different methodologies and measures which, in turn, will lead to a more consistent and coherent research base.

The final major area of development is in the area of training at three distinct levels. First it will be important to ensure that health psychology courses or their equivalent can be routinely introduced as part of undergraduate training in psychology. While this does appear to be happening in the United States (see earlier chapter by Dorsel and Baum), there has been relatively little movement in this direction elsewhere even though undergraduates do seem very interested in the general area. Thus a major task for health psychologists is to promote their discipline as an integral part of undergraduate training.

To increase the likelihood of good future research and to create the possibility of a professional status for health psychology, coherent postgraduate training at the Masters and Doctoral level must be initiated. In doing this, many issues and questions will come into focus. For example, should such courses be primarily aimed at producing researchers or should they be geared more to developing practitioner skills? Similarly, should the focus of such courses by mainly be primary prevention at the community level or should equal weight be given to work involving people with health problems in treatment settings? Clearly good courses must incorporate all these themes and approaches in order to equip future health psychologists to meet a broad range of challenges. However the immediate priority is to establish a strong research base in the discipline and one upon which any future practical applications can be based with confidence. The earlier chapters by Cynthia Belar and by Stan Maes and France Kittel have also considered these issues.

In planning future training initiatives, it is vital not to overlook the training of other health professionals in health psychology (see earlier chapters by Helen Winefield; John Christensen and Wendy Levinson; Hal Swerrison and Peter Foreman). Health psychology cannot exist in isolation from other branches of health care and health research. Moreover, many of the most ambitious research programs will inevitably involve collaboration with medical or nursing colleagues on the one hand and other biomedical researchers on the other. Effective teaching for these other groups will certainly not be achieved by offering a few one-off lectures in their training courses. It will be important to make full use of the insights from work on adult learning (e.g. Cross, 1982) in order to build on the experiences of these other groups and to bring about changes in their models of health and illness and hence in their perception of the role and value of health psychology. This is not a trivial task nor is it one which should be ignored since the resultant changes in knowledge and attitudes should serve to facilitate the progress of our discipline.

CONCLUSION

At present, the knowledge base of health psychology is still too limited and its methodologies are not sufficiently coherent or developed. Future developments should be responsive to social needs and to priorities in medicine as well as aimed at strengthening the discipline itself. If future work can succeed not only in providing valid accounts of the reol of psychological factors in health and illness but also in establishing good training at all levels, then the future is likely to be as exciting and productive as the recent past.

References

Amir, D. (1987) Preventive Behaviour and Health Status among the Elderly. *Psychology & Health,* **1,** 353–377

Cohen, F (1987) Measurement of coping. In S. V. Kasl and C. L. Cooper (Eds), *Stress and Health: Issues in Research Methodology,* Chichester: John Wiley.

Cross, P (1982) *Adults as Learners: Increasing participation and facilitating learning,* San Francisco: Jossey Bass

Elder, J. P., Abrams, D. B., Beardin, P. A., Carleton, R. A., Lasater, T. M., Lezieh, M., Peterson, G. S., and Schwertfeger, R. (1988). Behavioural community psychology and the prevention of heart disease: community level application of the Pawtucket Heart Health program. In W. Gordon, J. A. Herd and A. Baum (Eds) *Perspectives on Behavioural Medicine, Volume 3: prevention and rehabilitation.* San Diego: Academic Press.

Fallowfield, L. (1990) *The Quality of Life: the missing Measurement in Health Care.* London: Souvenir Press.

Howard, J. (1989) Exercise and physical fitness in the maintaining of health. *Paper presented at the Third European Conference on Health Psychology,* Utrecht, The Netherlands.

Hunter, J. R. W. (1984) The expert medical computer. In M. Yazdani and A. Narayanan (Eds), *Artificial Intelligence: Human Effects,* Chichester: Ellis Horwood

Leventhal, H., Meyer, D and Nerenz, D. (1980) The common-sense representation of illness danger. In S. Rachman (ed), *Medical Psychology,* Vol. 2., New York: Pergamon press.

This paper is based on the latter part of a recent overview paper by the author (Weinman, 1990).

Marteau, T. and Johnston, M. (1987) Health psychology: the danger of neglecting psychological models. *Bulletin of British Psychological Society,* **40,** 82–85.
Rigby, R., Brown, M., Anagnostou, P., Ross, M. W. and Rosser, B. R. S. 1989). Shock tactics to counter AIDS: the Australian experience. *Psychology and Health,* **3,** 145–160.
Schwarzer, R. and Leppin, A (1989) Social support and health: a meta-analysis. *Psychology and Health,* **3,**(1) 1–16.
Sherr, L. (1987) An evaluation of the UK Government Health Education programme on AIDS. *Psychology and Health,* **1,** 61–72.
Temoshok, L. (1990) Applying the biopsychosocial model to research on HIV/AIDS. In Bennett, P., Weinman, J. and Spurgeon, P. (Eds) *Current Developments in Health Psychology,* London: Harwood
Weinman, J. Psychological aspects of prenatal diagnostic screening. In L. Schmidt (Ed), *Psychological Aspects of Stressful Medical Procedures,* Berlin: Springer in press.
Weinman, J. (1990) Health Psychology: progress, perspectives and prospects. In Bennett, P., Weinman, J. and Spurgeon, P. (Eds) *Current Developments in Health Psychology,* London: Harwood
World Health Organisation (1981) *Global Strategy for Health for All By the year 2000* Geneva: WHO

CHAPTER 15

HEALTH PSYCHOLOGY IN INTERNATIONAL PERSPECTIVE: A SUMMARY AND SOME THOUGHTS FOR THE FUTURE

MARY A. JANSEN, GERDA J. METHORST and AD J. KERKHOF

Department of Clinical, Health and Personality Psychology, University of Leiden, Leiden, The Netherlands

This article reviews the progress made by the field in its short history and attempts to look at developments which seem likely to occur as the field matures.

Recommendations are made for training of health psychologists in the future and a plea is made for international standardisation of health psychology training programmes at the Ph.D. level which incorporate research and clinical training. Health psychologists are further encouraged to take a more active public and political role in order to provide needed visibility for their work.

As George Stone and his colleagues said in their chapter entitled "Health Psychology in the 21st century": "An attempt to look into the future is, . . . at first intriguing . . . but . . . the intrigue turns to anxiety, with terror lurking not far away" (Stone, Weiss, Matarazzo *et al.*, 1987, p. 513). The present authors know these feelings well and will not try to replicate the insightful and far reaching predictions made by Stone and his colleagues. Rather, we will take a more simplified and focussed look at where the field of health psychology is now and at what may be in store for the coming years.

First a look at where we are. In most countries of the developed world there is decreasing reliance on the medical profession as the field from which solutions to health problems should come (Dana and May, 1986). There has always been some awareness that medicine could not account for all health problems but increasingly there is recognition that solutions to health problems may be found by seeking psychological and behavioral solutions. It is now widely accepted that 60–70% of visits to primary care physicians are for reasons that are behavioral in nature (Broskowski, 1981). As recognition of this has grown, there has been increasing acceptance of the role of life-styles, attitudes, values, and beliefs as factors which play a part in health and illness.

A second factor which has led to greater interest in the possible contributions of health psychology to the health care system is the escalating cost of health care which is evident in every country. Actual rates vary but in most developed countries health care accounts for 10–15% of the country's gross national product. Much of this can be attributed to rapid technological advances, the continued reliance on costly inpatient treatment, and high physician fees. As a result public and private financing bodies are looking much more closely at ways to control these costs. It is to be expected therefore that the work of health psychologists in prevention and interventions which reduce reliance on the medical system will become increasingly valued. Thus there is greater interest in the variables which influence the development of illness, and which may help or hinder the attainment of good health. The need for greater accountability and the realization that psychological interventions can lead to decreased health care costs (Cummings, 1985) producing an overall savings in health care has encouraged the work of health psychologists in both research and applied settings. These factors have also created a more favorable political climate for research by health psychologists and development of clinical interventions based on this research.

These trends coupled with the growing body of knowledge of the relationship between behaviors and health has lead to the rapid expansion of the field over the last 15 years. This is carefully detailed by Stone (this issue). While this rapid expansion has been good, we must be certain to insure that continued development is based on clear directions for the field rather than a "jump on the bandwagon" approach. Thus, direction is needed for future research, development of clinical interventions, and perhaps most importantly for training of future health psychologists.

Research

A vast amount of evidence has accumulated pointing toward the relationship between psychological and behavioral factors and health. The extensive work in the area of stress is one example which has dramatically increased our knowledge of the direct and indirect effects which stressors can have on health. Work in the area of psychoneuroimmunology and the relationship of stress to the immune system holds promise of shedding light on some of the most threatening and debilitating illnesses. Cancer, HIV, and coronary heart disease are three prime examples where continuing research by health psychologists is needed to sort out the mechanisms which contribute to development of the disease process and the ways in which these mechanisms can be changed or stopped. These crucially important health problems require sophisticated and integrated research methodology, a commitment to carrying out research over long periods of time, adequate resources, interdisciplinary collaboration, and an acceptance of the inevitable delay in publication of results which comes from such complex and lengthy research endeavors (Schwartz, 1982; Taylor, 1987).

Research is also needed to find ways to change the life styles and habits which contribute to ill health. Overeating, smoking, failure to exercise, abuse of alcohol and drugs, undue stress, poor nutrition, and "unsafe" sexual practices are major contributors to the development of illness. Though obviously bad for health, we have found it difficult to devise effective strategies for helping people to change these behaviors. More research is needed to find ways to motivate people to change their life styles and habits, especially when this frequently involves delay of immediate gratification in return for the promise of better health and greater longevity in the future.

A further need is to develop psychological models specific to health care which can be used by health psychologists as they design clinical interventions (Marteau and Johnston, 1987). Thus, a unique psychological knowledge base is needed built on the awareness of human beings as a psycho-biological organism, and recognizing the contribution of cognitions, e.g. attitudes, beliefs, and values, to the prevention of illness and promotion of health.

Clinical Interventions

In its short history clinical health psychologists have made enormous strides in developing intervention strategies to enhance health. These range from preventive programmes aimed at decreasing the incidence of chronic health problems, compliance regimens designed to increase treatment compliance, and rehabilitation interventions aimed at increasing quality of life following illness or accident, thus preventing relapse or more serious consequences. Some excellent examples of interventions which have already proven their worth both in terms of effectiveness and in terms of reducing medical expenditures, include technology for managing chronic pain (Fordyce, 1976), preparation of patients requiring surgery (Mathews and Ridgeway, 1984) and psychological help for patients requiring other noxious medical procedures (Burish and Lyles, 1979; Kaplan, Atkins and Lenhard, 1982).

The potential role that prevention can play in reducing the incidence and severity of health problems is receiving greater attention. As research results from studies carried out now produce the ground work for future clinical interventions, prevention programmes will take on even greater significance. In order to translate these results into practical programmes that will be effective, health psychologists will need thorough knowlege of health care systems, familiarity with media techniques, and a greater role in the political process. As health psychologists identify an increased number of links between illness and behavior, our ability to design effective and usable intervention strategies to prevent health problems will dramatically increase (Bloom, 1988; Rogers, 1983), and the public, including insurance companies and corporations will see these services as cost effective ways to hold down health care costs.

Public education is also becoming increasingly important as we learn more about ways to improve health and prevent illness. The role of health psychologists is growing in educating legislative bodies about the benefits of preventive activities, funding bodies about the need for research in behavioral factors linked to illness, insurance companies about the cost benefit of psychological interventions, and the public about ways in which psychological and behavioral factors affect health.

Every community has a vital interest in the health of its members and many communities have health planning councils. Health psychologists have a responsibility to be actively involved in such community health planning efforts. Our knowledge of risk factors, life styles and ways to modify the interactions between the environment and health, importance of prevention, etc., provides both an opportunity and a responsibility to take an active role in community planning activities where these affect health.

An Illustration

The dramatic increase in the number of people infected with HIV worldwide has made this one of the world's most pressing public health problems. Until a cure for the disease is found, or a way to prevent it from developing is discovered, changing behavioral practices is the only way to prevent the spread of the disease. As those most knowledgeable about changing behaviors related to health, health psychologists are challenged by the need to educate the public about the importance of changing sexual habits and behaviors, and the need to find effective ways to influence people to adopt new behaviors and practices. Given the known discrepancy between knowledge, attitudes, and behaviors, this challenge is a difficult one. In addition, clinical interventions designed to assist patients and families in coping with the illness are needed along with interventions aimed at changing society's attitudes and eliminating the stigma attached to the disease. Clearly health psychologists have a major role to play in shaping the world's response to, and efforts to cope with, HIV.

One cautionary note about the development of intervention programmes is needed however. A clear need exists to document the effectiveness of clinical interventions which health psychologists offer. This can only be done by sound empirical research which points to the usefulness of the interventions we use (Agras, 1982; Dunn, 1983). Promotion of unproven methods can be damaging because we will be open to criticism from other health professionals who may feel threatened by health psychology's increasingly important role in health care.

Stress management programmes are an example of an intervention which was developed before solid evidence existed for its efficacy. Although we have learned a great deal about the relationship between stress, psychoimmunology, the cardiovascular system and hypertension, we have little formal evidence for the effectiveness of stress management programmes in reducing the incidence of any of the major illness. While it is likely that stress management programmes will produce beneficial results, the field of health psychology can be endangered by making claims that it can not back up. We should try to provide information about the known effectiveness of interventions whenever possible.

Training

All of what has been said up to this point places a heavy responsibility on health psychologists. The needed research, clinical interventions and community outreach can only be done by highly trained and competent health psychologists. The knowledge necessary to carry out these activities and to play a major part in shaping the future health of the world's population can only be gained after an intensive and lengthy program of study.

We have seen in the article by Methorst, Jansen and Kerkhof (this issue), that a wide diversity exists in training programmes for health psychologists. Internationally, content and level of training vary widely, thus raising questions about the quality of training offered in some areas. Fundamentally and most importantly, the issue is one of quality. It is the contention of the present authors that health psychologists must be trained at the doctoral (Ph.D.) level in order to have the minimum knowledge and skills, to take on the crucial challenges facing health care in today's world. We further contend that only those trained at this level should be called "health psychologists" in order to avoid confusion and to clarify the roles and responsibilities of health psychologists versus those with less training.

Training for health psychologists should also encompass the full range of both research and clinical aspects thus producing health psychologists who are knowledgeable about all aspects of research, service delivery, and the interdependence between the two. Training at less than the Ph.D. level may be appropriate to prepare individuals to assist in research programs, to carry out designated clinical applications and techniques under close supervision, and to act as first line workers in primary care. But the critical work of the field of health psychology (i.e. setting research priorities and designing empirically sound methods to reach those priorities, delivering direct psychological services to individuals, families, and groups in the health care system, designing and testing clinical interventions and evaluating their effectiveness, and delivering needed public health education and community planning consultations) consists of tasks that only highly trained and fully competent health psychologists can and should perform. To attempt to delegate these responsibilities to individuals with less than these competencies is a disservice to them, to the public and to ourselves.

Although it is tempting to find reasons why such high standards cannot be met, training programmes must not compromise their curriculum or their standards in order to accommodate the needs of faculty, the wishes of students, or the desires of financing authorities which often attempt to dictate what will be taught in a given programme. The issue of quality training and standards for the field is critical because the reputation and future of psychology itself lies in our ability to produce health psychologists who can meet the challenges of the highly complex health questions facing us today. In an era where competition for funds and for recognition is growing among health professionals, poor research, lack of good clinical skills, and lack of documented intervention effectiveness, will meet with skepticism and criticism, and will put the entire profession of psychology at risk (Mahrer, 1983).

In the coming years, young psychologists will be attracted to health psychology because it offers the opportunity to develop a solid research base and effective clinical interventions which have a major impact on the health of the world's population. A profession with this kind of promise can attract talented and aspiring young professionals but only if they see the profession as one where their knowledge and training will prepare them to make a difference. We must not disappoint them by providing less than the needed level and content of training to allow them to meet these challenges. A final point is that international standards for educating and for credentialing health psychologists should be developed (and as quickly as possible) in order to increase the credibility of the field for the various publics, including the government, other health professionals, insurers, the media, and the lay public.

What Will We See in the Future?

The integrated research and intervention strategies discussed in this paper require collaborative professional models in order to achieve the necessary mix of psychological, social, and biological inputs. This has already begun to occur and will continue as the importance of behavioral factors in health becomes clearer. This collaboration between disciplines should enhance the respect that each profession has for the other and help to diminish the growing competition among health professionals (Jasnosky, 1985; Spring, Chiodo and Bowen, 1987). This coupled with the important role which psychologists now have in training physicians and other care givers will further enhance the importance of behavioral factors in health (Davis and Butcher, 1985; Weinman and Medlik, 1985).

We are already beginning to see a greater influx of psychologists into the corporate world and away from strictly public services. As our intervention strategies become more reliable and the cost benefit ratios of providing psychological interventions is demonstrated, a greater demand for health psychologists will be seen in private corporations, in political circles deciding on future health legislation, and in privately financed insurance benefit programmes.

In poor areas the stresses encountered are different and of considerably greater magnitude. These include unemployment, poor nutrition, poor sanitation, high rates of illness and inadequate medical facilities, poverty, hard labor, war, excessive drug use and often lack of information about simple measures to improve health and quality of life. These stressors have been shown to be associated with increased psychological and physiological problems (Kasl and Cobb, 1970; Krantz, Grunberg and Baum, 1985). Although the stressors are different in many ways and the conditions under which they occur are vastly different, the applications of psychological research can have a great impact on the lives of people in poor areas. We can help to alleviate some of the effects of these stressors by teaching individuals better ways to cope and how to live more healthily, helping them to achieve greater control over their lives, thus mediating the effects of stress, and potentially increasing their quality of life and life expectancy.

The Cuban System—A Model for Health Psychology?

Reports from psychologists who have visited Cuba have indicated that the role of health psychologists in the Cuban health system is unique (Garcia-Averasturi, 1985; Kristiansen and Søderstrøm, this issue; Marin, 1985) because of the national recognition given to psychological variables in all aspects of health, and the national support for promoting health through incorporation of psychological principles and techniques at all levels of the health care system. It is reported that psychologists play a key role in the educational system thus instilling the value of a healthy life style in children.

These interesting reports deserve further study and point to principles which health psychologists in other countries may wish to work toward as health psychology develops around the world.

So, What Do We Do Till The Doctor Gets Here?

Although health psychologists will become much more in demand and a greater recognition of their important role will follow, health psychologists need to inform other health professionals and the public about their work and about its potential benefits. Many things depend on this assertive promotion, including increased funding for research, funding for development and evaluation of intervention strategies, funding for needed training programmes and the resources necessary to support such programmes, and recognition and government support for national and preferably international training and credentialing standards.

To some, these recommendations may seem far fetched, or even undesirable. To others, they may seem like good ideas, but hardly feasible. We believe that health psychologists can and should take a more active role publicly and politically in promoting the important role of behavioral factors in health and the critical role of psychologists in identifying these factors and helping people to achieve better health. Health psychologists, trained in clinical applications and in scientific methods, know how to translate research into practical applications which can help people to live healthier lives. To do less than this is to do a disservice to the public and to the profession of psychology. To do less will also prove to be a costly mistake in years to come as resources dwindle and competition increases for research funding, for full insurance coverage for clinical and prevention services, and for training programmes.

References

Agras, W. (1982). Behavioral medicine in the 1980's: Non-random connections. *Journal of Consulting and Clinical Psychology,* **50**, 797–803.

Bloom, B. (1988). Topical review: Primary prevention and the partnership of clinical, community and health psychology. *Journal of Primary Prevention,* **8**, Spring, 149–163.

Broskowski, A. (1981). The health—mental health connection: An introduction. In A. Broskowski, E. Marks and S. Budman (Eds), *Linking Health and Mental Health Services.* Beverly Hills: Sage.

Burish, T. and Lyles, J. (1979). Effectiveness of relaxation training in reducing the aversiveness of chemotherapy in the treatment of cancer. *Journal of Behavior Therapy and Experimental Psychiatry,* **10**, 357–361.

Cummings, N. (1985). Saving health care dollars through psychological services. *Congressional Record—Senate,* Volume 131, 85, 8656–8659. Washington, DC: U.S. Government Printing Office.

Dana, R. and May, W. (1986). Health care megatrends and health psychology. *Professional Psychology,* **17**, 251–255.

Davis, H. and Butcher, P. (1985). Sharing psychological skills. *British Journal of Medical Psychology,* **58**, 207–216.

Dunn, R. (1983). Psychology and health care. *Canadian Psychology,* **24**, 89–95.

Fordyce, W. (1976). *Behavioral Methods in Chronic Pain and Illness.* St. Louis: Mosby.

Garcia-Averasturi, L. (1985). Community health psychology in Cuba. *Journal of Community Psychology,* **13**, 117–123.

Jasnosky, M. (1985). Introduction—The Zeitgeist for health psychology. *American Behavioral Scientist,* **28**, 439–450.

Kaplan, R., Atkins, C. and Lenhard, L. (1982). Coping with a stressful sigmoidoscopy: evaluation of cognitive and relaxation preparations. *Journal of Behavioral Medicine,* **5**, 67–82.

Kasl, S. and Cobb, S. (1970). Blood pressure changes in men undergoing job loss: A preliminary report. *Psychosomatic Medicine,* **32**, 19–38.

Krantz, D., Grunberg, N. and Baum, A. (1985). Health psychology. *Annual Review of Psychology,* **36**, 349–383.

Mahrer, B. (1983). The education of health psychologists: quality counts—numbers are dangerous. *Health Psychology,* **2**, Supplement, 37–47.

Marin, B. (1985). Community psychology in Cuba: A literature review. *Journal of Community Psychology,* **13**, 138–154.

Marteau, T. and Johnston, M. (1987). Health psychology: the danger of neglecting psychological models. *Bulletin of the British Psychological Society,* **40**, 82–85.

Mathews, A. and Ridgeway, V. (1984). Psychological preparation for surgery. *In* Steptoe, A. and Mathews, A. (Eds), *Health Care and Human Behaviour.* London: Academic Press.

Rogers, R. (1983). Preventive health psychology: An interface of social and clinical psychology. *Journal of Social and Clinical Psychology,* **1**, 120–127.

Schwartz, G. E. (1982). Testing the biopsychosocial model: The ultimate challenge facing behavioral medicine? *Journal of Consulting and Clinical Psychology,* **50**, 1040–1053.

Spring, B., Chiodo, J. and Bowen, D. (1987). The social-clinical-psychobiology interface: Implications for health psychology. *Journal of Social and Clinical Psychology,* **5**, 1–7.

Stone, G., Weiss, S., Matarazzo, J., Miller, N., Rodin, J., Belar, C., Follick, M. and Singer, J. (1987). Health psychology in the twenty-first century. *In* Stone, G., Weiss, S., Matarazzo, J., Miller, N., Rodin, J., Belar, C., Follick, M. and Singer, J. (Eds), *Health Psychology: A Discipline and a Profession.* Chicago: University of Chicago Press.

Taylor, S. (1987). The progress and prospects of health psychology: Tasks of a maturing discipline. *Health Psychology,* **6**, 73–87.

Weinman, J. and Medlik, L. (1985). Sharing psychological skills in the general practice setting. *British Journal of Medical Psychology,* **58**, 223–230.

INDEX

E